© Copyright 2019 by Michelle Coles Jorgensen.

All rights reserved. This book or any portion thereof may not be reproduced or used in any manner whatsoever without express written permission of the author except for the use of brief quotations in a book review or scholarly journal.

First Printing: Independently Published, 2019

ISBN: 9781793012449

Layout and design by Julie Larsen

Dedication

Dedicated to my family for their unfailing support.
To my husband Steve, and my children Jens, Josh, Luke and Liza.
Your crazy wife and mother couldn't do it without you!

smiles@totalcaredental.com

Dr. Michelle Coles Jorgensen
DDS, FAGD, TNC, CNAS

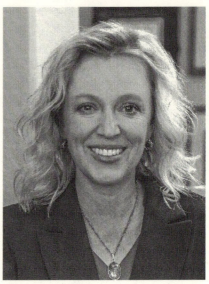

Dr. Michelle Jorgensen is an author, speaker, teacher, biologic/holistic dentist, and health and wellness provider. After practicing traditional dentistry for 10 years, Dr. Jorgensen became very sick. Through her own journey to return to health, she discovered she had mercury poisoning from drilling out mercury fillings for her patients without protection. She was concerned that there may be other health-threatening materials or procedures in dentistry, and this concern led her to the Biologic/Holistic Dentistry field.

For the last 10 years she has been paving the way in Biologic/Holistic dentistry, learning from pioneers all over the world. She has created the Total Care Dental Way, a patient CARE centric, health focused method for treating dental and over all health. Patients from around the world seek out her care, and come to Total Care Dental to have their health restored.

She has received certifications as a Therapeutic Nutritional Counselor, a Certified Nutritional AutoImmune Specialist, and is currently enrolled in a program to become a Board Certified Traditional Naturopath. She completed a Holistic Dental Mini-Residency, and is pursuing ongoing training from *Swiss Biohealth* in Switzerland and Costa Rica.

Dr. Jorgensen also teaches and coaches groups of dental professionals across the country who come to learn from Dr. Jorgensen at her Total Care Academy. Her goal is to change the way dentists look at health. She started and hosts a study group of Alternative Care Practitioners, where they teach each other and collaborate together for better patient care. This group includes Chiropractors, Naturopaths, MDs, Nurse Practitioners, Energy Workers and more.

A prolific writer, she has authored hundreds of blog posts and articles about dentistry, health and nutrition. She is interested in all areas of health and teaches classes to the public on topics ranging from *How to Raise Cavity-Free Kids* to *Fermenting Foods for Health*.

Since founding Total Care Dental in 2001, her dental practice has helped over 20,000 patients in Utah and the U. S. Dr. Jorgensen and her team have been awarded the *Dental Team of the Year* and the *Dental Practice of the Year* at the prestigious *Crown Council Member's Choice Award*. They were also selected as *Best in State in Utah* for multiple years.

When not at work Dr. Jorgensen is busy with her husband, four children, and her own mini-farm, where she loves to grow, harvest and preserve her own food. She loves to read and has a huge library of books on homesteading, gardening, natural health, herbology and so much more.

Healthy Mouth, Healthy You! – Holistic Dental Guide – Whole-body Health Starts in Your Mouth

Table of Contents

Forward- Robyn Openshaw, GreenSmoothieGirl.com 2

Introduction- Michelle Jorgensen, Total Care Dental 5

What You Can Expect from this Book- 8

Chapter One- What is a Holistic Dentist? 10

Chapter Two- What Teeth are Made of 16

Chapter Three- What Causes Cavities 19

Chapter Four- Clean the Outside 25

Chapter Five- Nourish the Inside 34

Chapter Six- Clean Up Past Problems 62

Chapter Seven- Fix the Mouth to Heal the Body 84

Chapter Eight- The Gum and Overall Health Connection 93

Chapter Nine- Heal what's Possible 111

Chapter Ten- Protect Your Body and Health 119

Chapter Eleven- Improve Your Smile 129

In Conclusion- 132

Quick-Start Guide to Holistic Dental Care- 133

Resources- 134

References- 137

Index- 151

Forward

In 1998, having learned that amalgam fillings were highly toxic, I went to a conventional dentist and had him remove them and replace them with white porcelain fillings. He couldn't fit a dental dam in my mouth, so he abandoned that idea. He used no specialized equipment, and drilled many metal fillings out of my mouth, potentially exposing both me and him to hazardous gases and metal fragments. I needed two root canals in a matter of several years after that.

In 2012, I went to a biological dentist for the first time, having learned that they offer options to toxic dental practices like amalgam fillings and root canals. He told me that my two root canals had "failed," and that I needed to extract both teeth and have zirconia implants replace them. I underwent a 5 ½ hour surgery with my mouth propped open wide. When I woke up, with a TMJ problem I'd never had before, I was handed a bill for nearly $20,000 for 17 procedures I didn't know I had signed up for, including replacing my fillings a third time that I'd had redone many years earlier.

This was the beginning of a long saga in which I learned a great deal about dental practices, and the wide disparity in the way various "biological dentists" think and practice. I learned, from interviewing many dentists, that there is no widely accepted definition of what a "biological dentist" is, and that the field is new enough that techniques are evolving, and not as "time-tested" as a patient might like.

Biological dentistry seems to be a term for a broad range of services provided by a dentist who has decided to provide less-toxic procedures and materials to repair (and clean) teeth. Some of them also provide all the conventional services they learned in dental school. Some take extremist positions, refusing to do any root canals, and some even refuse to place implants or refer patients for that procedure.

I bought a bunch of books by doctors, dentists, and attorneys on the thorny subject of conventional versus "biological" dentistry. I blogged on *GreenSmoothieGirl.com* about my dental saga and my evolving education, but quit talking about it publicly when the problems I was experiencing became so personally devastating that I needed to deal with it privately rather than publicly.

I discovered many things I wish I had known earlier. I had simply taken my dentist's word for it.

Failed root canals, teeth drilled on too many times, questionable implants—these are just some of the procedures that can (and have, in my case) "gone wrong" due to ignorance. The frustrating thing is, I read several books and many online reports and thought I knew more than I did. I am quite certain I read more than 99 percent of my fellow patients, but I was still grossly underinformed.

If I've learned one thing, it's to study the issue to the bottom before spending thousands of dollars, risking my dental health, and undertaking procedures for which there may be alternatives.

The fact is, in my miserable, three-year saga that totaled well over $30,000 in dental bills (out of pocket, since I am a self payer), I was paying the piper for the massive amounts of sugar I ate in my first 30-plus years of life. Americans want movie-star teeth, while eating more sugar than any pancreas, or any mouthful of teeth, were ever meant to handle. Perhaps we cannot, as the old saying goes, have our cake and eat it, too.

However, as discouraging as that may sound, information is empowerment. I believe you can start at a very high place of enlightenment if you are armed with a great overview of the body of knowledge in dental health. After all, you are reading this because you have teeth, and you'd like to keep them, and you'd like them to look good until you're old.

While compromises may need to be made, and no solution is necessarily perfect, you should know the pros and cons of your choices—preferably well before you face those choices.

I have now been the patient of several biological dentists. I have been friends with Dr. Michelle Jorgensen for several years and have watched her consume volumes of information, studying alternatives to the techniques she was taught in dental school and had practiced for many years. It was clear to me that she had propensity towards a holistic approach to health, as she had followed *GreenSmoothieGirl.com*, and my *12 Steps to Whole Foods* course, for years. She has a spectacular garden and feeds her family whole plant foods in a committed way I have rarely seen.

She truly "walks the walk." Plus, she was voraciously studying all the controversies in dentistry, wanting to do right by her patients. Early in her career, she started to experience health problems that she now feels were related to the heavy metals and chemical exposure in her work. She had the classic symptoms of heavy metal poisoning. This–and a desire to help her patients–led her to a commitment of providing her patients with accurate information and actionable alternatives.

When I felt Dr. Jorgensen had made a significant shift, I signed my family on as her patients. I have been consistently impressed with her quality of care and her ongoing open mindedness and quest for knowledge on the many controversies in dentistry. I'm also impressed with the quality of care and outcomes we have received.

She is also willing to tell us where she doesn't know the answer, because "the jury is still out" on some issues in biological dentistry. While it may be frustrating that some questions are still unknowns, I am skeptical of some of the "experts" writing on this topic who have ardent, committed stands on issues in which the field has insufficient longitudinal data or conflicted data. I appreciate her humility in presenting her synthesis of the methods and data, while allowing for some people's choice of traditional methods. To me, this is part of being a responsible practitioner.

Our conversations about the dental stories from *GreenSmoothieGirl* readers, and her patients led her to want to educate people as quickly and effectively as possible. Few seem to want to read the fat books on dentistry that we both have read! I hope you enjoy the condensed information Dr. Jorgensen will share, and that you are enlightened and empowered by more knowledge about your options.

Sincerely,

Robyn Openshaw, Green Smoothie Girl
GreenSmoothieGirl.com

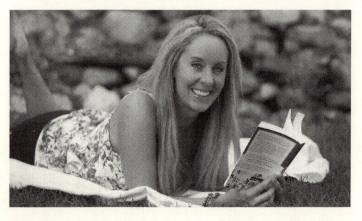

Introduction

I come from a family of dentists. That's just what we do. My father has been practicing for nearly 40 years, and because he loves dentistry, it has been his hobby as well as his profession. Three of my younger brothers and I watched this passion and decided to follow in his footsteps.

I was trained to perform traditional dental procedures in school, and continued my education over nights and weekends after graduating. I couldn't get enough! I too grew to love this profession and thought I would work for forty years, just like my dad. Then my health issues started.

It was nothing big at first, just some digestive issues. I though it probably had something to do with what we were eating. As a busy mom of four young kids, I realized our entire family could benefit from some changes. I started reading and researching, and we started slowly. We began having a green smoothie for breakfast. I had to pay my kids to drink them for the first month, but the habit stuck. I was blown away at this whole new way of eating and looking at food. It wasn't just about calories or yumminess, it was about how we wanted to fuel our bodies. Again, I couldn't get enough!

I continued to learn and implement things over time and started to see changes. All of us noticed a difference in our health. The kids didn't get sick anymore, my husband dropped ten pounds, and most of my digestive issues went away. Things were looking up, but it wasn't all better.

I continued having some nagging digestive issues, and, more of a concern, I was having numbness in my right arm and hand. Many doctors and chiropractors later, no one had any answers for me. Then my memory started to slip. I've always had an excellent memory, and I felt like my brain was filled with fog. What was going on??

I needed to find the answer, so I continued to learn about nutrition, and eventually ventured into alternative health. I became a Therapeutic Nutritional Counselor to learn more. I tried muscle testing, energy work, biofeedback, acupuncture, infrared saunas, supplements, homeopathy, essential oils, massage, super foods... and on and on. No changes. It was tough to get out of bed each morning, let alone put on a happy face for 20-30 patients each day. I was depressed, couldn't remember things, had no energy and was ready to quit dentistry.

As a last effort, I decided to look into holistic dentistry. Perhaps I could slow down and do nutritional counseling instead of dental procedures. It would be easier on my body. I found a successful holistic dentist and shared my story with him. He sighed and said, "You sound just like me ten years ago. Have you looked into mercury poisoning?"

I didn't know what he was talking about. I hadn't placed a mercury filling in over 10 years (the profession calls them "amalgam" or "silver", but any non-gold metal filling is 50% mercury). He told me the problem isn't when you place the filling, it's when you remove it. When a dentist removes an old mercury filling, it sends mercury vapors into the air. I had been removing multiple mercury fillings every day for the last 10 years, without any sort of protection. I had a very probable case of mercury poisoning.

After a heavy metal test, I found I did indeed have very high levels of mercury. Finally, I had an answer! I started a lengthy detox program, and slowly felt my energy and my memory return. I wondered what other harmful things were going on in my dental practice every day. I realized I had come a long way in my understanding about nutrition. Now it was time for me to transition my dental practice into a place where I could restore health, not just fix teeth.

True to form, I couldn't get my hands on information quickly enough. I bought every Holistic dental book on Amazon and tried to read them all in a week! I learned about programs and bought videos. I studied research articles and started trying things in my practice. Most of my patients liked this change in focus, and it felt good. I started to enjoy dentistry again!

Through all of this study, I learned two things. First, there are a lot of myths and controversial subjects in dentistry, and most people are either far on the alternative side or far on the traditional side. I couldn't find many that ventured toward the middle. You might ask why I want to be in the middle. Well, what I found through years and mountains of research was that some dentists were too strident, too enraged, too frustrated to be objective. They have a "they are out to get us" mentality that I don't relate to, ignoring all that is good in the traditional dental model. Others in traditional dentistry ignore strong evidence that practices we accept as "standard of care" are outdated, and have proven to be harmful, or even potentially toxic or dangerous.

The second thing I learned is that the information is too technical and way too lengthy for most people to read. Some of the books are over an inch thick. Even I didn't want to read them, and I'm a dentist! I decided I wanted to provide an easy to read, easy to follow, honest guide to dentistry. These are not the results of research studies in an isolated lab, these are my results from day to day practice with people just like you.

This book is very personal to me, because the things I will share saved my health and my career. I hope they can help you too.

Sincerely,

Dr. Michelle Jorgensen, DDS, FAGD, TNC, CNAS

totalcaredental.com

smiles@totalcaredental.com

What You Can Expect from this Book

When I began to write this book, I thought long and hard about what would be most important to include. I wanted to focus on how to never have a cavity again, how to provide a mouth-friendly diet for your family, and how to avoid the problems in traditional dentistry (and medicine.) On the other hand, I also needed to educate readers on the detrimental and even sometimes dangerous practices and products in dentistry, and how to get out of the dental mess they may already be in. I realized I had to include some of both, and keep with my goal of providing explanations that are simple to understand and recommendations that anyone could start tomorrow. No easy task!

I also had to decide where I should stand on the spectrum of traditional and alternative therapies. There are radical outliers on both sides, and I knew talking to the fringes would help some, but not many. So my approach is to meet people where they are, and present the good in all therapies–if they are truly good. I will be honest about my opinions, and if I don't know if something is helpful or harmful, because the research is simply not there yet, I will tell you exactly that.

I know you are all busy, and as patients and friends have told me, "Most of the other books on this topic overestimate our interest in dentistry!" I may want to read all of the holistic dental books on Amazon, but you probably don't, and I don't blame you. I am going to give you the *Reader's Digest* version of holistic dentistry–all the most important and useful information, without the extras that just fill lines and take time. If you are the kind of person who loves the extras, please look for the list of articles and information at the end of the book.

Here is a sneak peek at some of the questions and controversies that will be addressed in this Guide to Whole-Body Health and Wellness:

1. What is a holistic or biologic dentist?
2. How do teeth get cavities?
3. How can I make my teeth cavity-proof, naturally?
4. How can I clean up old, toxic dentistry like silver fillings and root canals?
5. How can these old dental problems be causing or contributing to my chronic disease like heart disease or cancer?
6. Why do I need to clean my mouth to protect my whole body, and how are they interrelated?
7. How do I fix new problems in the healthiest way possible?
8. Which dental problems can heal, and how can I make it happen?
9. How can I have a healthy, dazzling smile?

   ...and much more!

Chapter One: What is a Holistic Dentist?

Most traditional dental experiences are similar. You visit the dentist every six months, or when you get around to it. At that visit, they polish your teeth, scrape the crusty stuff off, then the dentist comes to complete a cursory exam. You sit tensely, waiting for the verdict. Did you brush enough? Can they tell you never floss? Maybe you really did inherit your mom's bad teeth.

You're told about the cavities that need to be filled, the teeth that need "crowns" or perhaps even "root canals," and you glumly sit and listen. As you prepare to leave, you're given a toothbrush and floss, maybe told to use the floss a little more often and scheduled for another "cleaning" appointment in six months. You return to have the recommended dental work completed, pay the bill and continue doing everything the same as in the past, cursing those bad tooth genes.

What's missing in this scenario? So MANY things! Why did you get the cavities? How can you prevent them in the future? How will that crown or root canal affect you? Are there alternatives? Are there things you can do with your dental habits that that could have a huge impact on your overall health?

Disconnected Dentistry

Unfortunately, dentistry has followed modern medicine right down its disconnected, reductionist path, separating body parts and processes. You need an ENT for ear problems, an OB/GYN for women problems, a dentist for tooth problems... there is a doctor for every little part and piece of our bodies. Somehow we've forgotten that it's all the same body. When was the last time a dentist talked to you about the relationship between your mouth health and your overall health?

The other big issue in modern Western medicine and dentistry, is that the focus is almost entirely on symptoms, instead of the source or cause of the problem. Why did you get that cavity? Does it have to do with what you eat or if you are getting enough nutrients from your food? Do your hormones affect your teeth? How long is that filling going to last and what is it doing to your tooth and body? Who knows? No one talks about it. This leads to a never-ending loop of exams, fillings, crowns, root canals, surgeries and dental fears that never even address the root of the problem.

How did we get this way and are the tides turning? The answer is yes and no. The tides are certainly not turning in the education of dental professionals. I did not have one nutrition class in dental school. I was trained to place and remove mercury containing fillings, without one thought or concern about the toxicity of that metal. Root canals and fluoride are the standard of care. I've talked with new graduates and they report the same.

However, if you look outside of the dental schools, you will see a lot of talk about alternative dental care and treatment ideas. This information and interest is coming from concerned consumers like you. You are frustrated with the lack of preventive care in dentistry. You are concerned about the possibility that your dentistry is making you sick. You want dental professionals to help you with your HEALTH, not just your TEETH, because you realize they are connected, even if they don't.

A holistic or biologic dentist works to breaks this loop. He or she focuses on the treatment of the whole person, rather than just the symptoms of dental disease. That is a lot to tackle, and each practitioner does it in a little different way based on their training and experience, but the focus will always be on something bigger than just your dental problem.

I must say it is about time! Renowned German Physician Dr. Reinhard Voll estimated that nearly 80% of all illness is related entirely or partially to problems in the mouth.[1] According to the National Institutes of Health, Americans spent $33.9 billion out-of-pocket on CAM (Complimentary and Alternative Medicine) practices and products. If we can receive alternative care for medicine, it's about time the same is available for dentistry.

The Whole-Body Connection

Most of the research about the connection between whole-body health and dental health has occurred outside of dental education and practice. It's an example of the common saying, "You can't see the forest for the trees". The field of dentistry is so focused on the details of treating TEETH, they can't see that that treatment of the teeth has affected the entire BODY! Some of the most outspoken doctors about this tooth-body connection are cardiologists and Cancer centers.

Dr. Thomas Levy, MD, JD has written a book in 2017 titled *"The Hidden Epidemic."* It is full of long-standing scientific research pointing to the overwhelming health effects of dental infection. He says, *"The vast majority of the adult population of the world has at least one significant* tooth infection. Yet, these teeth nearly always go undiscovered and are rarely addressed. **Nevertheless, it is these teeth, along with infected tonsils and infected gums that cause the vast majority of heart attacks and cases of breast cancer."**[1]

Some of the diseases that have been shown to be connected to dental infection are:

- Heart Disease
- Cancer
- Alzheimer's disease
- Anemia
- Diabetes
- High Blood Pressure
- Inflammatory Bowel Disease
- Metabolic Syndrome
- Osteoporosis
- Pregnancy complications
- Prostatitis
- Pulmonary disease
- Hearing loss
- many more...

In his 2011 book, *Whole-Body Dentistry*, Dr. Mark Breiner, DDS laments that, *"This year millions of adults and their children will needlessly suffer a broad range of preventable illnesses. Less serious conditions, like excessive fatigue and headaches, may go unnoticed or will be incorrectly attributed to aging or stress. Hundreds of thousands of individuals will develop more serious conditions ... These people will become ill for no apparent reason. But more often than not, there is an underlying issue that triggers these people's illnesses, and that issue is often found in the mouth."*[2]

Based on over 40 years of research, renowned German Physician Dr. Reinhard Voll estimated that nearly 80% of all illness is related entirely or partially to problems in the mouth.[2]

These findings and statistics would surprise almost any health practitioner, but particularly dentists, including me. I realized just how serious these dental-health connections are when I reached out to alternative cancer treatment centers for patients that needed their care. They informed the patients and I that they would not see them to treat their cancer until all their dental conditions had been treated and resolved. They have learned the cancer treatments will not be effective while chronic infections remain in the mouth.

I am fascinated to hear that patients don't get this information from their cancer doctors, heart doctors, or even their previous dentist! Why aren't more health professionals talking about this with every patient?

We have been trained to treat dental conditions in a mechanical "drill and fill" method. If there is a hole in a tooth, it needs to be filled. We have not been trained to look for the sources or causes of the problem, or to look deeper into how these dental problems could be affecting the rest of the body. This is new territory for most practitioners. We have not been trained to look at the forest, because we spend so much time looking at the trees.

Dental Training

Like most other graduate schools, the training received in dental school is basic and very traditional. The schools make sure their students are able to perform dental procedures before they graduate. They learn to diagnose dental problems, clean teeth, fill teeth, crown teeth, root canal teeth, pull teeth and replace teeth. Some dentists never complete another day of training after dental school, so their practices are centered on "fixing" teeth. That's all they have been taught to do. It is up to the individual dentist to invest their time and money into learning more.

If you are looking for a dentist that will do more than just fix your teeth, there are certain things to look for. If their website has nothing more than information on pretty smiles and fillings, you may want to move on.

SOME QUESTIONS TO ASK YOUR DENTIST

1. Is it a "Mercury Free" *and* "Mercury safe" dental practice? These are two different things. "Mercury free" simply means the dentist does not place mercury containing fillings, and thankfully, quite a few dentists fall into this category now. "Mercury safe" means that all mercury is handled safely, and when removing old mercury fillings, you and the dental team will be protected. Make sure the office is MERCURY SAFE.

2. Do they have a special protocol for removing mercury fillings? To handle mercury safely, the office will have a mercury removal protocol including physical protection for you and the dental team during removal. This should include rubber dam, high volume suction and skin and airway protection, amongst other things. The office should also have a protocol for you to follow nutritionally to prepare your body to excrete the metals after removal.

3. Do they use digital xrays? X-rays have been and will continue to be a concern in medicine and dentistry, but they are safer now than ever before. With the introduction of digital xrays, the radiation used for an xray is drastically reduced. Xrays are essential in proper diagnosis, but should only be done digitally to keep you safe.

4. What is their position on fluoride? Fluoride has had a very controversial journey. It does make a tooth *stronger*. However, there are very undesirable side effects of fluoride usage that are often ignored. Fluoride should be used sparingly and never ingested if possible.

5. Do they address nutrition in relation to dental health? The dentist has probably talked to you about not eating sugar... but that is the tip of the iceberg on how nutrition affects dental health. Nutrition can hurt or heal your teeth, bone and gums, and the entire dental team should all be able to guide you to a Mouth Friendly diet.

Michelle Coles Jorgensen, DDS, FAGD, TNC, CNAS

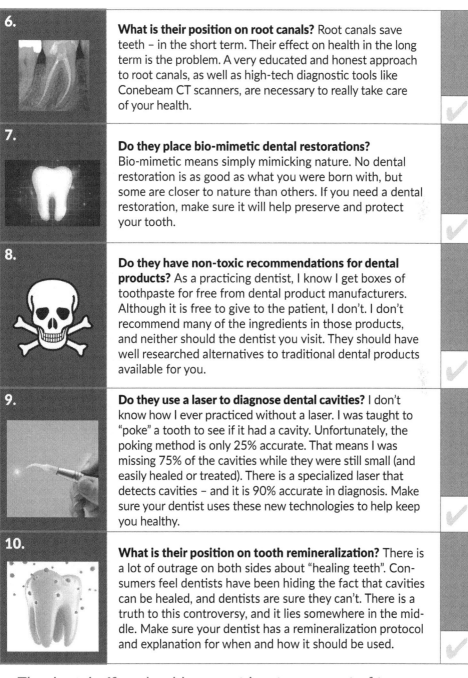

6. What is their position on root canals? Root canals save teeth – in the short term. Their effect on health in the long term is the problem. A very educated and honest approach to root canals, as well as high-tech diagnostic tools like Conebeam CT scanners, are necessary to really take care of your health.

7. Do they place bio-mimetic dental restorations? Bio-mimetic means simply mimicking nature. No dental restoration is as good as what you were born with, but some are closer to nature than others. If you need a dental restoration, make sure it will help preserve and protect your tooth.

8. Do they have non-toxic recommendations for dental products? As a practicing dentist, I know I get boxes of toothpaste for free from dental product manufacturers. Although it is free to give to the patient, I don't. I don't recommend many of the ingredients in those products, and neither should the dentist you visit. They should have well researched alternatives to traditional dental products available for you.

9. Do they use a laser to diagnose dental cavities? I don't know how I ever practiced without a laser. I was taught to "poke" a tooth to see if it had a cavity. Unfortunately, the poking method is only 25% accurate. That means I was missing 75% of the cavities while they were still small (and easily healed or treated). There is a specialized laser that detects cavities – and it is 90% accurate in diagnosis. Make sure your dentist uses these new technologies to help keep you healthy.

10. What is their position on tooth remineralization? There is a lot of outrage on both sides about "healing teeth". Consumers feel dentists have been hiding the fact that cavities can be healed, and dentists are sure they can't. There is a truth to this controversy, and it lies somewhere in the middle. Make sure your dentist has a remineralization protocol and explanation for when and how it should be used.

The dental office should score at least seven out of ten on this questionnaire if they are really whole-body and health focused. Don't settle for less.

Chapter Two: What Teeth are Made of

Teeth are alive! They work just like every other organ in your body. They respond to your nutrition, your health, your care or your misuse. My favorite example to explain the anatomy of a tooth is to compare it with an M & M type of candy. The outside layer is like the hard candy coating and the inside layer is like the soft chocolate center. While not anatomically correct, it's an easy way to think about a tooth! Also, if you've ever had a pocketful of M&Ms on a hot summer day, you know that even that M&M is vulnerable at times.

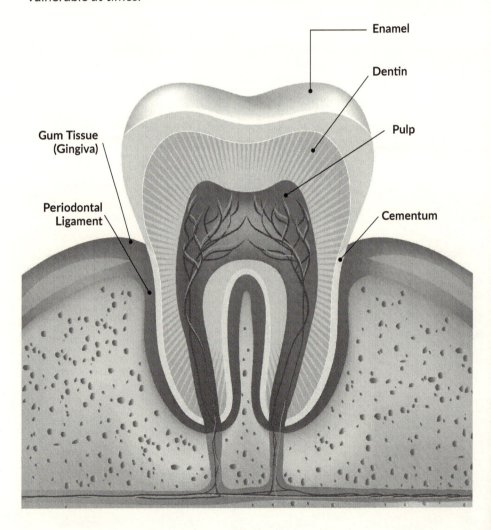

Enamel

The outside "hard candy coating" layer is called the enamel. It is the part of the tooth you can see, and it is made of calcium and phosphate, combined into crystals called hydroxyapatite. Those crystals are stacked up, side by side, but have small spaces between them where fluid can flow. The fluid can flow from the outside in, or from the inside out. The more minerals in these crystals, the stronger and more impenetrable they are.

Dentin

The first part of the "soft chocolate center" is called the dentin. This is a mineralized layer that supports the enamel. It is softer and darker in color. If you were to look at it under a microscope, you would see that dentin has miles of tiny tubules, running from the inside of the tooth to the enamel. In one molar, there is a football field worth of these small tubules.

Pulp

The pulp chamber is in the very center of the tooth. This chamber contains nerves, blood vessels, cells, and connective tissue. This is where nutrients are passed from the bloodstream to the tubes in the dentin. This is also where sensation in the tooth comes from.

Connective tissue cells line the outside of this pulp chamber. These cells are called odontoblasts, and each cell lines up with one of those tubules in the dentin. They have a long arm that extends up into that tube, pumping fluid, nutrients and transmitting pressure changes to the nerve below. These cells also continue to rebuild dentin throughout the life of the tooth.

Cementum

The enamel covers the exposed part of the tooth but ends where the gums begin. The root is instead covered with a much softer, mineralized collagen coating called cementum. This layer ends at the very end of the root where the nerves and blood vessels exit.

Periodontal Ligament

Thousands of ligaments extend out from this cementum to the bone surrounding the tooth, connecting the tooth to the bone. These ligaments slightly suspend the tooth, allowing for shock absorption as your teeth are used. These ligaments are called the periodontal ligament.

Gum Tissue

The tissue lining your mouth and extending up to the edge of each tooth is called gingiva and is only one cell thick. This thin layer is your defense against the 400-plus microbes, as well as toxins and infection that may enter your mouth. This is the only barrier between your mouth and your bloodstream. There is a tight collar of this tissue surrounding each of your teeth, and this collar is important in keeping your tooth and your body healthy.

As I continue to demystify dentistry for you, you will find that this simple explanation of teeth will make our answers easier to understand. Mark this section as you may want to reference it often. [1]

Chapter Three: What Causes Cavities

Let's tackle a big controversy right now: What causes cavities? You know the standard answer. Brush your teeth and stop eating sugar and you won't get cavities. This isn't wrong, but it's not the whole story.

First of all, let's talk about what a cavity is. Your mouth is a veritable battlefield, with acid and bacteria as the enemies to strong teeth. If your mouth is acidic (from diet and overall health issues), that acid pulls minerals out of the enamel, leaving it weak and vulnerable. If enough minerals are pulled out (called demineralization), bacteria can travel through the enamel to the dentin, and the dentin becomes infected. Once the infection starts, it is called dental caries or a "cavity."

There has been an upward trend in caries (cavities) since the 1990s. An article from the Centers for Disease Control in 2016 states that, *"Although dental caries are largely preventable, they remain the most common chronic disease of children aged 6 to 11 years and adolescents aged 12 to 19 years. Tooth decay is four times more common than asthma among adolescents aged 14 to 17 years. Dental caries also affects adults, with 9 out of 10 over the age of 20 having some degree of tooth-root decay."* [3]

There has been an increase in decay, while people in the US spend over $20 billion on dental care annually[3] Toothpaste commercials saturate the airwaves, and we have at least two generations of people who have been "educated" on what to do to prevent cavities. Poor dental hygiene alone can't be the cause for all of these cavities. Despite more spending on dental care than any other time in history, dental health is as bad or worse than it has ever been. Something is missing.

Decided by Vote

In the 1940's, at a meeting of the *International Association of Dental Research*, the attendees wanted to end the debate over the cause of cavities. There were three heavily researched theories that were debated, along with others. These theories were:

THE ACIDOGENIC THEORY	
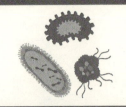	Bacteria in your mouth are fond of sugar. When they eat sugar, they produce acid as a waste product. This acid dissolves the minerals in your tooth and you get a cavity.[4]
THE DIET THEORY	
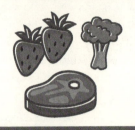	Dr. Westin Price was a dentist that was frustrated with dental decay. He took 10 years to travel the world, looking for groups of people that had good dental health. He studied those people and found consistent, common nutritional reasons for healthy teeth and mouths.[5]
THE HORMONE THEORY	
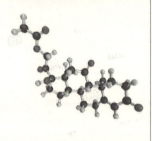	Dr. Melvin Page also researched dental decay, and found that there is an internal fluid flow in teeth that naturally helps the tooth stay clean and healthy. This flow is controlled by hormones. When the hormones are not balanced, this fluid flow reverses and brings toxins into the tooth rather than out.[7]

After evaluating the data from many research studies on the topic, the majority felt that the **Acidogenic Theory** (sugar + bacteria) was the most correct. This was adopted as fact, and that decision holds strong today, despite evidence to the contrary.[4]

I don't think they were wrong in 1940, but I don't think they were completely right either. I believe there are multiple factors that contribute to tooth decay, and my years in practice have confirmed this.

I often examine the teeth of an entire family at the same time. I'll see a wife that recently gave birth, and she has five new cavities. Her husband secretly confides that he hasn't flossed a day in his life, and he's never had a cavity. Their children are a mixed bag—some with cavities and some without. They eat the same food and have similar dental care. Why the difference in decay?

There are volumes about this, but I'm going to give you a simple version that will help you know how to prevent cavities in the future.

The Role Sugar Plays in Tooth Health

Sugar on the teeth is not what causes cavities. The sugar feeds certain damaging bacteria, and these bacteria create acid. It is this acid that dissolves and pulls the minerals out of the enamel, leading to cavities.

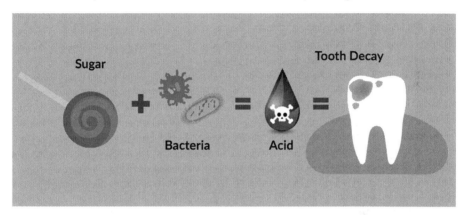

We all have bacteria in our mouths, and some live in that sticky plaque that makes your teeth feel "fuzzy". We need bacteria to protect us, but some also cause problems. You can reduce the number of harmful bacteria (more on this later), but you can never get rid of all of them. If that plaque stays on your teeth, the bacteria multiply. If you feed them their favorite food–sugar–they will create acid which will dissolve your enamel. As you learned above, if enough minerals dissolve, you will get a cavity.

The Umbrella Effect and Cavity-Resistant Teeth

As I said, this is not wrong, but it isn't the entire story. If it was, the husband in the previous example would have more tooth decay than his wife. When you're using an umbrella, the water beads up on the surface and doesn't soak in because of the tightly woven fabric of the umbrella. It is water resistant. If your tooth enamel is full of minerals, it becomes "cavity-resistant" in much the same way. In fact, if your tooth enamel is strong and healthy, what you put in your mouth–sugar or not–will not have as much effect.

My younger brother taught me the truth behind this. During his teenage years, he had new-fangled "white braces" put on his teeth. He rarely brushed, so those white braces became orange braces, green braces–the color matched the meal. Funny thing was, he never got cavities around those braces. If cavities are always caused by bacteria and plaque on your teeth, he would have had a mouthful. What protected his teeth?

> *"If you feed your body and teeth the right nutrients, your tooth will protect itself."*

His teeth were cavity-resistant. His enamel was healthy. This has everything to do with those miles of tubes in your teeth. Your teeth are fed from the inside through blood vessels in the center pulp layer of the tooth. Those blood vessels send nutrients to the pumping cells, the odontoblasts, which pump them through the dentin tubules to the enamel above. If you feed your body and teeth the right nutrients, your body will protect itself by using those nutrients to strengthen the teeth. What are those nutrients? You will find this information in much more detail in *Chapter Five– Nourish The Inside*.

Hormones and Tooth Health

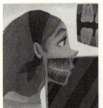

- Lauren visited my office for a second opinion. While away at college, she saw a dentist for a cleaning and was told she had 16 cavities. Mom insisted she see me—sure the other dentist was trying to get more money from her unsuspecting daughter. I took new dental x-rays and told her my findings. She didn't have 16 cavities—she had 17.

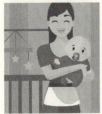

- Sharon never had a cavity until she had children. The first baby led to five cavities and fillings, the second to another four and a toothache, and she was nervous about what a third pregnancy would do to her dental health. Despite taking meticulous care of her teeth, she continued to have dental problems until she visited my office.

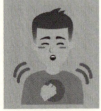

- Jerry always had great teeth, until he had a heart attack last year. Soon after that, he started noticing dark, sensitive areas along the gumline of his teeth. He came for a checkup, and I diagnosed those dark areas as rapidly growing cavities.

All of these people have something in common—they have tooth decay that isn't caused by sugar. Women who are expecting, growing teenagers and people that are suffering from chronic illness all share increased risk for tooth decay. What is the connection? Hormones.

Dr. Melvin Page and other researchers found that when our hormone-secreting glands are out of balance, teeth start to decay. Let me explain how this works. We already learned about the tubules inside your tooth and the cells (odontoblasts) that live at the end of each of those tubes. Those odontoblasts pump fluid up and through the dentin and enamel. This fluid is like lymphatic fluid, and it cleans the tooth from the inside out. It repels plaque and bacteria, food and debris on the tooth. It's like having a toothbrush on the inside. Amazing, isn't it? [8]

This fluid flow is directed by the parotid gland, a saliva gland near your cheeks. This communicates with the hypothalamus, an area in your brain highly affected by hormones. When hormones are out of balance, this system reverses. The fluid draws the bacteria and debris into the tooth. This leads to tooth decay.

There are natural causes for hormonal imbalance, including pregnancy and teenage puberty, menopause and male hormone decline. There are also unnatural causes like prescription drugs, environmental hormone disrupters (some foods, EMF wavelengths, etc.), and having a diet high in white sugar and flour. Chronic disease also affects the balance of all the regulatory pathways in your body, including your hormones. If you are in one of these risk categories, you must do more to prevent cavities. [6]

Main Causes of Tooth Decay Revealed

To summarize, there are many things that lead to tooth decay, but here are the three main players:

1. The **bacteria** on your teeth consume sugar and leave acid behind. This acid dissolves and weakens the enamel, letting more bacteria in.
2. If your tooth is weakened because of **nutritional deficiencies,** the tooth will be more susceptible to this acid attack.
3. If your **hormones** are out of balance, your tooth's inner fluid flow reverses and it will be difficult to prevent decay.

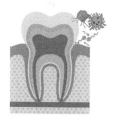
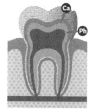
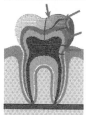

Do not despair! If you have one or more of these tooth challenges, keep reading! We will discuss how to predictably remove the bacteria off the teeth, strengthen the teeth through diet, and balance hormones to make your teeth resistant to this hormonal challenge.

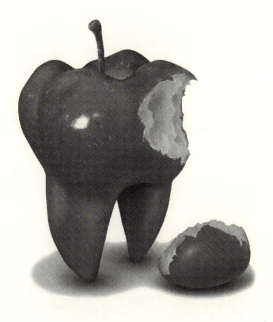

Chapter Four: Clean the Outside

If the first attack on your teeth comes from bacteria and the acid they produce, let's talk about how to keep those bacteria off your teeth. You've heard it before–your mom probably told you at least 100 times to "Brush your teeth!" She was right. But do you know HOW to brush your teeth, and WHAT to use on that brush? Let's start there.

Nothing Secret to Clean Teeth

As I started to transition my practice to a holistic-based dental practice, I had my team read books about holistic dentistry with me. When we got to the sections on tooth care, my hygienists were frustrated. These books were claiming to teach the "secrets" about preventing tooth decay and gum disease.

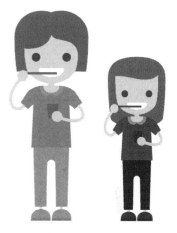

Why were they frustrated? Well, the recommended techniques were not secret. They were not even revolutionary! In fact, your grandmother may have been using some of them. Second, the procedures were lengthy and required multiple steps, a variety of products and a lot of commitment.

Don't get me wrong—if you want to spend 30 minutes a day caring for your mouth and teeth, I couldn't be happier. But in my 20 years of practice, I've found very few people who are willing to do that (myself and my family included). To help you, I've gleaned ideas from many different techniques to create a simple, every day routine that anyone can do.

What Do You Use?

I'm all about simple. If you have to look for it, buy it, and replace it when it runs out, the likelihood that you will use it decreases substantially. So, I will send you to your kitchen cupboards for most of what I recommend.

Finally, hold your breath... I'm going to go way out on a limb on this one and say, **"You only NEED to clean your mouth completely ONCE a day."** Notice I changed it up. There is a difference between brushing your teeth and cleaning your mouth. Let me explain:

Once a day – **the right way** – mouth cleaning

Step 1: Clean at the Right Time

After a long day of eating and drinking and dealing with stress and environmental toxins, your body, particularly your mouth, is acidic. If you start to brush your teeth when your mouth is acidic, you will brush your tooth away. Literally. Remember those enamel crystals and what happens to them in an acidic environment? It's just like that M&M in your pocket on a hot summer day.

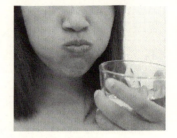

You need to pay attention to when you are cleaning. You should not clean your teeth immediately after a meal (your mouth is acidic from the food). Wait at least 15 minutes for your mouth to balance. Also, you should never clean your teeth immediately after an acid attack like throwing up or drinking a very acidic beverage (i.e. soda).

If you've had a hard day, haven't eaten well, and if your mouth feels very dirty, it's a good idea to balance the acidity (measured by pH) in your mouth BEFORE cleaning to protect your teeth. A simple sea salt rinse will do just that. How? The salt makes your mouth slightly more alkaline, in preparation for your cleaning.[1]

Sea Salt Rinse

Ingredients:
2 t. sea salt or Himalayan salt
2 cups nearly boiling purified or distilled water
1 pint-sized glass jar with a tight fitting lid
small 1 oz. cup for each person

Combine the hot water and salt in the jar. The hot water will help the salt dissolve completely. Wait until it is room temperature to use. Pour 1 oz. into a glass and start to rinse. Rinse vigorously with the salt rinse for 30 seconds, making sure to pull the rinse over all the surfaces of your teeth. Spit it out and rinse with plain water if desired.

(Make this up ahead of time in quarts if you would like. Keep it sitting next to your sink to use. Remember – simple!)

Step 2: Brush your Teeth AND Gums (2 ½ Minutes)

There are three things we need to clear up here:
1. What type of brush should be used.
2. What toothpaste is best to brush with.
3. How to brush, and for how long.

What type of toothbrush?

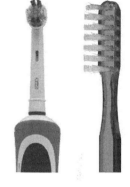

There are some essential things to look for in a brush. *#1—Soft, round-ended bristles.* There are only two purposes for a firm bristled brush: To clean your toilet or scrub oil off your driveway. Anything firmer than soft is too damaging to your teeth.
#2—The head should not be more than 1 inch long. I prefer something even smaller. You have to be able to maneuver it around your mouth.
#3—A handle small enough to hold easily in your hand.

My favorites are a manual Bass toothbrush with soft bristles, or an Oral B electric toothbrush.

What toothpaste should you use?

This one is a loaded topic. I'm sure you've heard that nine out of ten dentists recommend you use *(insert brand that spends the most for advertising here)* toothpaste. Remember, a large percentage of dentists have education limited to dental school training, which is not holistic in any way. We are taught to repair damaged teeth, and few of the treatments taught are "natural" or focused on being body-friendly.

Well, I'm the one out of ten dentists that doesn't recommend you use any of the big brand tooth care products! In fact, there are few I do recommend, and here's why.

Do you know what those commercial toothpastes have in them? [2]

Propylene Glycol: Used in antifreeze
Triclosan: An antibacterial agent that affects your good bacteria and hormones
Artificial colors: Potential allergen
Fluoride: Evidence of neurotoxicity (more on this in a later chapter)
Ethanol: Alcohol that dries your mouth and may cause oral cancer
Artificial sweeteners: Cause GI problems
Detergents *(like sodium laurel sulfate):* Cause gums to bleed and become "leaky"

Trisodium Phosphate: a commercial cleaner that is extremely alkaline
Glycerine: Coats the enamel so teeth can't remineralize
Carbomer: Very acidic thickener

If you've ever watched children brush their teeth, you know they swallow more toothpaste than they spit out. You do too. I don't want my family or me swallowing any of these things! Another problem is that the detergent in the toothpaste makes it foam. That foam quickly fills your mouth and you have to spit. Some think that spitting means they are done brushing. More foam = less brushing.

So what should you use instead? I've searched far and wide to find a toothpaste that is easy to find, tastes decent and actually has some beneficial ingredients. I've found one that almost fits the bill, plus I've come up with a recipe for homemade toothpaste that completely does.

Earthpaste, from Redmond Clay Company is my current winner in the toothpaste category. My kids will even use it, despite it being brown. My homemade paste uses almost the same ingredients, with a few small changes. The base is Calcium Bentonite Clay Powder. The benefits of this clay have been known for centuries—it is only recently that we've forgotten these important things. Clay can absorb and remove toxins and remineralize and polish teeth, all things we are looking for!

Dr. J's MouthPaste Recipe

2 T Bentonite Clay—Absorbs toxins, chemicals, and heavy metals.
 Releases minerals (calcium). Helps cells get oxygen. Alkalizes.
2-3 T Boiled Water, cooled
2 T 10% Nano-Silver—Potent natural antibiotic that slows bacteria growth in the
 mouth but doesn't kill healthy bacteria you need for good immune function.
4 drops Tea Tree Oil—Topical antiseptic, anti-bacterial, anti-fungal
 treatment. Reduces infection.
15 drops Peppermint or Lemon Essential Oil—Promotes healthy function of the
 digestive, immune, and respiratory systems.
5 drops Liquid Stevia—Comes from the leaf of a South American shrub.
 Very sweet but doesn't cause cavities.
Pinch Real Salt—Pulls toxins from the cells and alkalizes the mouth.
Instructions: Mix all ingredients together and store in an airtight container for use.

Other tooth care products that I recommend can be found in the appendix section about Resources and Products.

How to brush[3]

Last but not least-how should you brush your teeth? Remember my dentist father? He loves to brush. He has a few toothbrushes in the side pocket of his car door, and he often brushes while driving (I know, not too safe, but it's hard to fault him for brushing!). I learned the proper technique while watching him every day as he drove me to school.

Start with just a very small amount of toothpaste (the size of a pea). The toothpaste isn't the most important part here, and if you use too much you will have to spit it out. Start brushing in the back of your mouth. I always start on the bottom right, tongue side. If you want to add more toothpaste as you brush, if you have have sensitive teeth or want to remineralize your teeth, do it after you spit.

1. Position the brush in the middle of the tooth, but aim the bristles at a 45 degree angle down toward the gums and move it gently back and forth over 1-2 teeth. Think about polishing that plaque off right at the gumline.

2. After the back and forth motion at the gumline area, sweep the brush upward across the rest of the tooth. You are bringing that plaque to the top.

3. Repeat for the next tooth in line. You should move from one tooth to the next, brushing each one, and then sweeping up on each one.

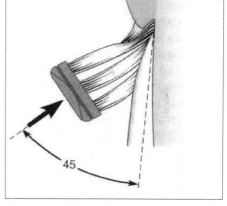

Bass brushing technique

4. Take about 30 seconds to clean all of one section in your mouth. For me, that would be all the back sides of the bottom teeth. Spit everything out (you're spitting out the plaque you removed, but you don't need to rinse at this point).

5. Move to the next section. Now I do the front sides of the bottom teeth. Do the same along all of those teeth for 30 seconds. Spit.

6. Repeat for the other two sides-fronts of top teeth and backs of top teeth. 30 seconds each and spit at the end of each side.

7. You now have any remaining plaque sitting on the tops of the teeth. Brush the chewing surfaces for 15 seconds each, top and bottom. (This is where children get the most cavities, so make sure they don't skip this step!)

If you did your math right, that takes 2 ½ minutes. I usually take close to 4 minutes, but that's just me being a little obsessive! If you have a dedicated 2 ½ minutes, that will do the trick. You have now removed plaque from the gums and the teeth, stimulated the gums and cleaned the chewing surfaces to prevent cavities. Good job!

Step 3: Clean Your Tongue (30 sec.)

This one is very personal to me. When I was in college, I had a very serious boyfriend share with me that my breath wasn't always so great. This killed me! I was going to be a dentist and I thought I knew about fresh breath. I was wrong. If you've ever worried about your breath, this one is for you! I also learned my problems were digestion-related and we will get to that later in the book.

Look at your tongue. You will see that it is not so smooth. I tell patients it is like a shag carpet! In fact, it is covered in tiny grooves and potholes. All of those bumpy surfaces are great at collecting plaque and mucous. Yep, it's that same stuff that makes your teeth fuzzy and your nose stuff up. The longer it stays there, the smellier it gets.

I used to brush my tongue very well, or so I thought. Then I was introduced to a tongue scraper. I used it one night, after brushing my tongue, and was appalled to see all the gunk coming off. Right there and then I became a true-blue tongue scraper, and I will never go a day without it.

It also helped me solve one of my dental mysteries. There is a dental condition called *geographic tongue*. I had it. It's where smooth patches move around on your tongue, you experience soreness from acidic foods and even when eating. There is no official known cause, but I have my own thoughts about what it's from. When I started scraping my tongue every night, my tongue would bleed because of this condition. After consistent use, the bleeding stopped and the patches went away

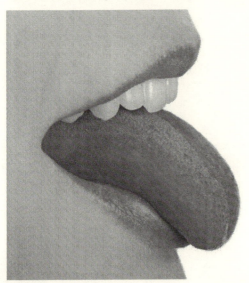

completely. I have been free of geographic tongue (and hopefully bad breath) for over 10 years. I now know it's from plaque, mucus and yeasts living on the surface of the tongue. Yuck!

My favorite tongue scraper is from Philips called Breath RX. Another that is good is from the Oolit company. *(See Resource section)*

How to:

Bend the tongue scraper toward you, grooved side down, making a "u" shape. Put the round part of the "U" as far back on your tongue as possible, while sticking your tongue out. Scrape forward against the surface of your tongue. You will see gunk on the grooves in the scraper. Rinse and repeat. Keep doing it until there is no more gunk coming off. Time needed: 30 seconds.

Step 4: Clean Between the Teeth (1 min)

I know what you're thinking. Here we go- the floss lecture. Well, it's going to be very different than you've ever heard before. There is a reason you need to clean between your teeth. Plaque and food squeeze in there too, and if it never gets cleaned, well, you're setting yourself up for possible tooth issues.

Here's what you haven't heard before. I would rather you not floss. You heard that right! First, you probably aren't flossing anyway, and second, I believe it opens up pockets for plaque to get into if you routinely push the gum away from the tooth with floss.

I do care that you clean between your teeth, and there are many ways to make that possible. Choose one–that's all I ask!

Clean-in-between menu of choices

- *Water Irrigator* (Waterpik)– this shoots water all round and in between your teeth. It's great if you have alot of dental work or braces.

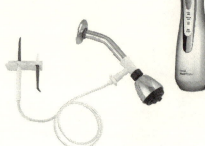

- A Shower Flosser– This is my personal favorite. It is a Waterpik that attaches to your shower head. You divert water to the flosser and get to spend more time in the shower while cleaning your teeth (and it's great at cleaning the grout on your shower tile and the gunk out of your wedding ring!)

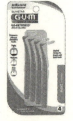

- *Christmas Tree cleaners* (Go-Betweens)– this isn't what they are called but they look like miniature Christmas trees. The fuzzy part cleans between the teeth.

- *Toothpicks*– Now you don't have an excuse at all. Everyone can use a toothpick.

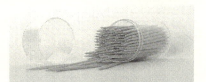

Step 5: Final Rinse (30 sec.)

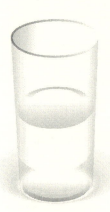

You have your choice of rinses here, but don't choose a traditional mouthwash!! They have a high alcohol content, and actually end up drying out your mouth and causing more bacteria to grow and more bad breath.[4] Some good choices:

- **Plain water**
- **That same salt water you started with**
- **Dr. J's Clean and Heal Rinse**

> **Dr. J's Clean and Heal Rinse**
>
> 1 T baking soda
> 1 t sea salt or Himalayan salt
> 2 C water
> 2 T colloidal or nano silver solution
>
> Mix all ingredients in a glass jar. Use 1 oz to swish with after cleaning your teeth.
>
> *(You can make up a lot of this at a time as well to simplify life. It is good for 1 month or more.)*

Whew!— that sounded like a lot, but if you add it up, the cleaning takes five minutes. Give yourself two minutes to get the products out and put them away, and that makes seven. If you will take seven minutes a day to really clean your mouth, you may be able to eliminate tooth decay and gum disease in your mouth completely.

Why did I say seven minutes a day? Because if you do it right once, you only have to do it once. You read that right. I do all of this at night because it fits in my routine. If you prefer the morning, that works as well.

I confess, I do also clean in the morning–the morning breath alone motivates me to do that, but I don't do everything–I only brush. So, once a day, the right way and touch ups as you need them. That's it!

Chapter Five: Nourish the Inside

Let's go on a trip! Dr. Weston Price was a well-known and respected dentist in Ohio in the 1930s. He became concerned about the increasing amount of tooth decay, abscesses and crowded and crooked teeth he was seeing in his patients. He was particularly concerned about children. He had heard of native societies in other parts of the world with strong, healthy teeth, and he wanted to see for himself what they were doing to avoid dental problems.

Teeth around the world

He and his wife began traveling the world, studying traditional people and their diets. Over ten years' time, he visited isolated Swiss villages, Gaelic communities in the Outer Hebrides, indigenous peoples of North and South America, Melanesian and Polynesian South Sea islanders including New Zealand Maori, African tribes, and Australian Aborigines. Although the diets were all different from culture to culture, everywhere Dr. Price visited he found beautiful, straight teeth, little tooth decay, good bone structure and resistance to disease among the peoples who ate only their traditional diet.

His timing was perfect. There were still societies that were untouched by modern food, but not for long. In some communities, he found members of the same family eating in very different ways. In one family, the older brother ate the traditional diet of the area, and the younger brother had adopted a modern diet. This allowed him to see the true effect of diet. The two brothers had the same genetic makeup, and yet had different dental problems.

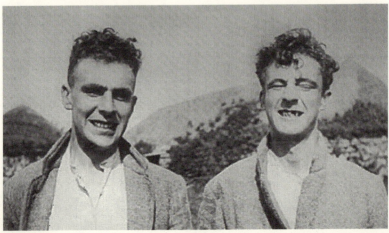

The value of the traditional diet

He found that people who started turning their back on their traditional diets did not have the same healthy teeth as those who had stayed true to how they had been eating for centuries. When they added processed and refined foods such as white flour, white rice, jam, canned foods, condensed milk, and sugar, they started having tooth decay and crooked teeth, and started suffering from degenerative modern diseases these communities had never seen before.[2]

His work is indisputable due to one key piece of evidence–he had a camera. He took rolls and rolls of pictures, documenting his findings in vivid detail. What did he find? What did these people eat that was so key to their health?

More nutrients = healthy teeth

Dr. Price found that the diets of these traditional people were very nutrient-dense. They contained vastly more vitamins and minerals than the American diet of his day,[3] and that Standard American Diet has been in steep decline since the 1930s. The difference would be even more pronounced today. Traditional diets provided at least FOUR times the water-soluble vitamins, calcium, and other minerals, and at least TEN times the fat-soluble vitamins than people were getting in America at the time. Although different societies were eating different *foods* (some were eating whale blubber and others butter from grass-fed cows), the constituents of those foods were the same.[4]

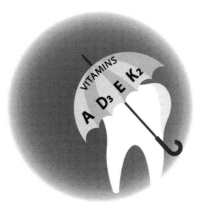

Is this the missing piece? I think it's one of them. Remember the concept of the water-resistant umbrella? Dr. Price figured out how to have strong, decay resistant teeth–and what he found surprised even himself. He conclusively showed that a major contributor to tooth decay and chronic disease in modern civilization is a lack of nutrients in our modern diet. Today's scientists have validated what Dr. Price's findings

What are those nutrients that are essential to healthy teeth? Fat-soluble vitamins A, D3, E and K2.

Fat soluble vitamins help absorb essential minerals

Without getting too technical, not all the vitamins and minerals you eat are able to get into the places they are needed. Imagine a key in a lock. Unless you have the right key, you're not going to get through that door, no matter how much you need to get through! Fat soluble vitamins are the right keys. They make it possible for your body to absorb minerals and use protein.[5,6,7]

As a biologic dentist, I am able to provide dental care for a lot of the alternative health care providers in my area. One nationally known speaker that promotes nutrition visited me to have her teeth cleaned. It had been many years since she had seen a dentist, and after the cleaning, my hygienist told me, "you really need to do an exam." I visited with my friend and patient for a few minutes and then started to examine her teeth. I was shocked. She had numerous dental issues, not the least of those being 10 cavities. I showed her what I was seeing, and we were both stumped. What had happened??

*I mentioned that she needed more minerals in her body to replace those lost from her teeth. She exclaimed, "I eat **tons** of minerals!" I know her personally, and she does eat tons of minerals. They had not been able to get into her teeth. Because her raw vegan diet had left her deficient in fat-soluble vitamins. She had been eating minerals, but they were leaving her system without being absorbed.*

What are these master key vitamins, and where do you get them? I don't like taking a hand full of pills in the morning, and my body doesn't like it either. I'd much rather get the nutrients I need from the food I eat, so I will share food sources. However, in today's commercial farming and factory processed meat world, it is increasingly difficult to get the vitamins and minerals you need from these foods, so I will give supplement recommendations as well.

Fat-Soluble Vitamin Roles and Sources

Vitamin A : Plays many roles

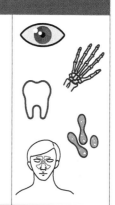

- Helps the eyes adjust to light changes.
- Important in bone growth and tooth development.
- Aids in reproduction, cell division and gene expression.
- Works to regulate the immune system.
- Keeps the skin, eyes, and mucous membranes of the mouth, nose, throat and lungs moist.
- Important antioxidant that may play a role in the prevention of certain cancers.

Food Sources for Vitamin A

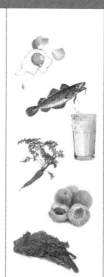

- The form that is easiest for your body to use is from animal foods—butter, milk, egg yolks, goat cheese, fish and liver. Two particularly rich sources are fermented cod liver oil and butter. You can use an Extra Virgin source of cod liver oil or a fermented version, but make sure your sources are clean and the oils are handled properly.[8]
- Some plants contain the antioxidant beta-carotene, which the body can convert to vitamin A. It is a little more difficult for the body to make this conversion, but it is a great plant source of the vitamin.
- Beta-carotene comes from orange or dark green fruits and vegetables. Examples are carrots, pumpkin, winter squash, dark green leafy vegetables and apricots.

Vitamin D3: Helps the body use calcium and phosphorous.

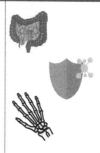

- Increases the amount of calcium absorbed from the small intestine, helping to form and maintain bones and teeth. This also prevents tooth decay.
- Plays a role in immunity and controlling cell growth.
- Children especially need adequate amounts of vitamin D to develop strong bones and healthy teeth.

Food Sources for Vitamin D3

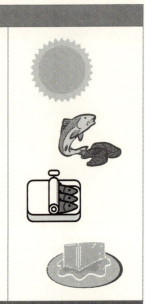

- The primary source of Vitamin D is the sun. You need to spend time in the sun, without sunscreen on, in order to have the effect needed to create Vitamin D in the body. The best times are between 11am–2pm for Vitamin D formation.

- Vitamin D is also found in oily fish (e.g., herring, salmon and sardines) as well as in cod liver oil, butter, eggs and liver.

Vitamin E: Benefits the body by acting as an antioxidant

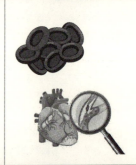

- Protects vitamins A and C, red blood cells, and essential fatty acids from being destroyed.
- Fights damage by free radicals that are created through chemical processes in our body. They neutralize these harmful substances.[10]
- Eating an antioxidant rich diet full of fruits and vegetables, lowers the risk for heart disease, cancer, and several other diseases.

Food Sources for Vitamin E

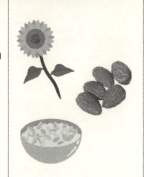

- About 60 percent of vitamin E in the diet comes from vegetable and nut oil (olive oil, almond oil). Watch out for oils high in Omega 6 Fatty Acids like Soybean, Canola, Corn, Cottonseed, Sunflower, Peanut and Sesame Oil.[11]

- Fruits and vegetables, grains, nuts (almonds and hazelnuts), seeds (sunflower) and fortified cereals.

Vitamin K2 : Enables cells to use Calcium	
• Works synergistically with Vitamin D3 to uptake calcium into cells[12] • Essential to remineralize tooth decay. • Particularly important in times of hormonal change such as puberty and pregnancy.	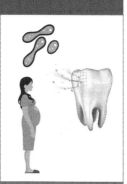
Food Sources for Vitamin K2	
• Raw dairy products have the highest concentrations of this vitamin. Butter oil, raw butter or ghee (clarified butter–you can make it or purchase it), and raw cream. • Fish, Eggs	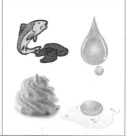

Patients that have heard about my approach to dental care often come to me for a second opinion. A common situation I'm asked to give an opinion on is the heart broken teenager that has just been told they have many cavities. These are the kids that have had good teeth, a few small cavities, but nothing significant. At their latest dental visit they are given the jaw-dropping news that their dental story has changed, and they now have 10, 15, even 20 cavities.

The parents are even more stunned, and their pocket books are feeling the pain as well. They come for a second opinion, and more often than not I confirm the findings. They usually do have that many cavities. The guilt-trip starts. "Aren't you brushing your teeth?? Are you drinking soda all day? What is going on?" Sometimes these are the reasons for the cavities, but often, nothing has changed in their diet or tooth cleaning. So why the cavities?

It's all about the nutrients! When a teenager is growing, there is a high demand for minerals that build bones. If they are not getting enough out of their diet or supplementation to supply that demand, the body will find them where it can. One of those supply houses of minerals is the teeth. The body needs the minerals, the body takes the minerals from the teeth leaving them weak and susceptible to tooth decay. Simple, sad story that is played out every day in dental offices around the country. The biggest problem is that most patients AND dentists don't know the source of that tooth decay, so the story continues.

Research is Valid for today

There is one fundamental difference between Dr. Price's research and dental research conducted today. Dr. Price did not set out to prove anything; he was looking for answers and didn't have any preconceived notions about what the answers might be. He had no agendas, no corporate backers, no theory he could manipulate the data to prove. He was unbiased. For me that gives complete validity to his research. I can't deny his findings.

His Book, *Nutrition and Physical Degeneration*[1] is nearly three inches thick! In addition, he published extensive research to support his findings in the book, including a two-volume work titled *"Dental Infections Oral & Systemic"* and *"Dental Infections & the Degenerative Diseases."* While most traditional dentists have never heard of Dr. Price, he started the holistic dentistry movement, and a small but growing number of dentists are adopting his research and developing new and more natural ways to treat teeth.

How to Eat to Build Decay-Resistant Teeth

Dr. Price found that the groups of people most resistant to tooth decay ate from the following food groups 2-3 times a day:[1]

- Dairy products from grass-fed animals
- Organs from fish and shellfish
- Organs of land animals

Think back to your diet over the last week. Have you had some fish and fish heads lately? How about liver? I'm guessing your diet, along with 80% of the rest of us, might be deficient in fat soluble vitamins and tooth building minerals.

I'm going to get on a small soap box for a moment. I love Dr. Price's research, and value what he learned. Unfortunately, it's not so easy to apply his recommendations directly to what we should eat today. Why? The food these indigenous populations were eating, and the food available to us today from conventional food stores, is not the same food.

When was the last time you had butter made from fresh cream, from cows fed spring-green grass at the edge of a glacier? Was the beef you had for dinner from a grass-fed happy cow that lived in a beautiful meadow with other happy cows? This is a problem, but we can do something about it.

Food that Really Feeds a Body

When I'm not at the dental office, you can often find me with my fingernails filled with dirt, flannel shirt and garden clogs on. I love to garden and work in the soil. And when I say soil, I mean soil. I add compost to my garden every fall, and all winter long the wonderful world of soil building microbes goes to town. By the time spring rolls around, that soil is full of nutrients, just waiting to fill my produce with good-for-me things.

Contrast that with modern day commercial farming. The soil is sterilized to avoid weeds and pests, killing all beneficial microbes in the process. Because those microbes aren't around to build the soil and feed the plants, the plants are fertilized with synthetic fertilizers to help them grow.[13] Think of the difference between a healthy athlete and one pumped up on steroids. The synthetic fertilizers don't add nutrients to the plants, they just make them grow bigger.

I also raise chickens and goats on my family mini-farm. Why in the world do I do that? Because when we eat the eggs and milk from those animals, we are eating what they eat. My animals happily munch on organic kale and collard greens, left over lettuce, cucumbers and squash. We even supplement with sprouted barley in the winter when fresh greens are scarce. We joke that our animals eat better than a lot of people!

Now I'm a realist and I know the large majority of people are not going to raise their own animals and most don't have access to fresh home grown organic produce. If you belong to that large majority, what do you do? This is one of my passions! You can find food that is full of nutrients, but you have to work a little harder to find it.

Where to Get Nutritious Food

One of my favorite sources of healthy, home grown food is online classifieds. Yes, I'm talking about Craigslist! You can often find local farmers that are selling their produce and animal products for much less than you will find from retailers. Times to look for these products are when they are in season. During bumper crop years, home growers are often willing to give away the produce if you provide the labor to harvest it.

What if you are nowhere near a farm? *The Environmental Working Group* publishes and updates a list every year called *The Dirty Dozen* and *The Clean Fifteen*. This list identifies the foods most and least likely to be contaminated with pesticides. Look at the *Quick Start Guide to Dental Health* at the back of the book for the online sources each year. Use this as your buying guide.

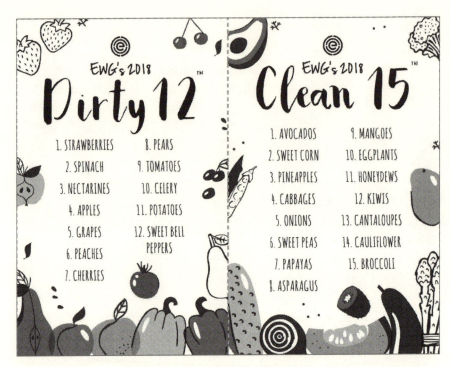

It may not be worth the extra dollars or effort to purchase organically grown varieties of the foods on the *Clean Fifteen* list. Go ahead and buy those at your regular grocery store. But please, go out of your way to find cleaner sources for everything on the *Dirty Dozen* list. When I saw strawberries topping the "dirty" list year after year, I vowed never to eat a non-organically grown strawberry again. That sounds snobbish, but I don't want to eat pesticides, and those strawberries will be very inferior nutritionally. I would rather eat a food that fills me with nutrients, than something that fills me with chemicals.

The Dairy and Bone Problem

There are two concerns with mass produced dairy products available today. The first concern is pasteurization. Milk is full of tooth-building calcium, but we need the enzyme phosphatase to absorb that calcium. When milk is pasteurized, it is heated to 165 degrees or more. This heating destroys phosphatase, along with important parts of other vitamins like Vit C and beneficial probiotics. Without the phosphatase, all of that wonderful calcium remains unavailable to you. This leads to deposits of inorganic calcium in places we don't want it, like tartar on your teeth, plaque in your arteries and stones in your organs (gall bladder and kidney are two common areas). You're drinking the calcium, but it can't get into your teeth and bones.[14]

The second problem with conventional dairy products has to do with the quality of the milk. Most milk, even organic milk, is from cows that are not raised naturally. Cows naturally eat grass, but in nearly every dairy in the country, 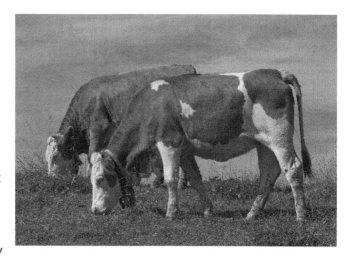 the cows are fed grains and other inexpensive food that are not part of a cow's natural diet.[15] The result is milk that is too sweet and lacking in nutrients. For example, Vitamin K2 is essential for tooth and bone health, but is only found in dairy products if the cow has been eating grass, not grain. Unless specifically labeled, you can assume that store-bought milk is from grain fed cows.

What to do about it

If grass-fed dairy is such a valuable source of fat-soluble vitamins and other minerals, how can we find it? Due to laws that are meant to protect us, unpasteurized raw milk can be difficult to find. There is a website called www.realmilk.com that can help you locate raw milk in your area. You may also find information at www.westonprice.org/chapters.[16]

My mom loves to tell a story about trying to feed me when I was a baby. If you've ever fed a baby, you've probably tried the split-spoon method at least once. You put something delicious on the front of the spoon, and something not so appetizing on the back, like applesauce and peas. You hope the babies' love for applesauce will distract them from noticing they ate a little peas too! My mom had to employ the trick in a little different way for me. She would put a green bean on the front of the spoon, and ice cream on the back. This is backwards from most babies, and I'm afraid I've been a little backwards about food my entire

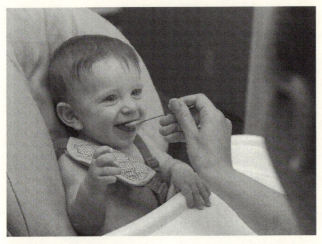

life. I didn't like ice cream, but I loved beans!

Dairy products have never been my friend. I've always felt lousy after eating them. So, for me, even raw milk isn't a great solution. If you look at research, you'll see that a lot of us do suffer from an intolerance to the sugar in dairy called lactose. We produce too little lactase, the enzyme necessary to break lactose down.[17] I know there are many of you who would prefer not to include dairy in your diet for this reason, or other, so how do we get the nutrients dairy products provide?

Fermented foods and their benefits

I have discovered fermented dairy products, which have changed my life and my health. These fermented foods have been staples of diets for centuries, as it was the only way to preserve dairy products in days before refrigeration. Their popularity had decreased when new forms of food preservation were discovered. However, new research is showing there are health benefits with these foods that can't be derived from any modern day food processing means.

I love fermented foods and have frequent Kombucha, Kefir, Raw Yogurt, Fermented Vegetables and Natural Yeast Breads in my home. Full of beneficial microbes, these foods not only taste great, but also help heal and protect your body. Here are some of the benefits:

1. Easier to maintain a healthy weight [18]
2. Reduced heart disease, Type 2 diabetes and overall illness [19-22]
3. Improved sugar handling and reduced sore muscles [23]
4. Anti-diabetic and Anti-obesity [13]
5. Helps with immune disease like IBS and Arthritis [25]
6. Improve mood and brain activity [26-28]

The fermentation process predigests the proteins in the food, such as lactose and gluten, helping make them easier to digest. It also fills the foods with beneficial bacteria that aid in overall digestion. This is why I can eat my homemade yogurt, kefir and cheeses. I now start my morning with a raw milk yogurt smoothie. My teeth are less sensitive, stronger, and healthier than ever!

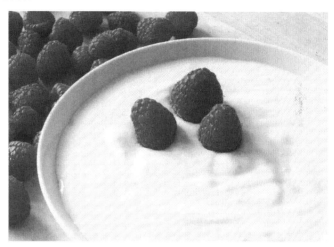

In summary, even though dairy is high in calcium, in it's non-fermented and pasteurized form, it isn't used well by the human body. Fermentation will transform this damaging food to something very beneficial, and raw sources will provide calcium that is usable. If you don't have either of these forms available to you, I believe you should leave dairy products out of your diet.

How much calcium do we really need?

Adults need 1¹/₂ grams per day of calcium. Some great sources are seafoods like salmon, clams and shrimp, broccoli, cauliflower, beet greens, nuts and olives. Green food sources are kale, bok choy and cabbage.[29] I'm not talking a few vegetables here. You need seven cups of kale to get that much calcium in one day. I hope you love kale! Greens are also the most bioavailable source of calcium.

One more caution–oxalates! All of the dark leafy greens have a high oxalic acid content. This acid binds to calcium and creates oxalate crystals.[30] This also makes the calcium unavailable to you. In order to inactivate the oxalic acid, you need to lightly steam the greens before eating them. Or you can add a calcium tablet to the cooking liquid. It will bind with the oxalic acid so the calcium in the food is available for you.

A woman was referred to me by her naturopath because she had a toothache. When she opened her mouth for an exam, I could immediately see why the tooth hurt. It had a porcelain crown on it, and was the only tooth hitting when she chewed. All of her other teeth were literally dissolving away in her mouth! I couldn't figure out why. She was healthy, athletic, had a great diet and took good quality supplements. I was stumped until I had her tell me her typical diet in detail.

She started off the day with a smoothie with greens in it. Lunch was a big salad, then dinner was veggies with a huge helping of greens. She was taking the advice she had been given to eat more greens, but she had taken it to the extreme. None of these greens were cooked, so they were full of oxalates. She was unwittingly depriving her body of calcium, and her body was taking the calcium it needed to survive from her teeth.

She had to have all of her back teeth rebuilt to the height of that one porcelain crown. It was a sad result of health recommendations taken to the extreme. Now she cooks her greens at night and eats a variety of healthy foods for the other meals. Her overall and bone health has also improved.

Bone broth

Bone broth is a hot topic these days, and it makes me smile! Although it's touted as a "new" health food, cooks have been making bone broth over fires for centuries. Bone broth is simply water infused with nutrients pulled from slow cooking marrow containing bones. Or in simpler terms, it's made by boiling bones in water for a long time. It has proven to be good at clearing congestion and as an anti-inflammatory food.[31]

I often cook a whole free-range chicken in my crockpot. (See recipe on the next page). We use the meat for 2-3 meals in the week, and the bones for broth.

Fall-off-the-bone Crockpot Chicken (makes 3 meals!!)

4 t salt
2 t paprika
1/4 t cayenne pepper
1 t onion powder
1 t thyme
1 t pepper
1/2 t garlic powder
1 large free range organic roasting chicken, thawed

1. Combine spices in a small bowl.
2. Remove any giblets or neck from the chicken (look on the inside and take out anything that looks like it doesn't belong!)
3. Rub spice mixture all over the outside of the chicken (I put it on a plate to do this, and dump the spices that fell onto the plate on top when it's in the crock)
4. Put chicken into the crock pot and cook on low for 7-8 hours. No liquid is needed—it will make its own juices.

My broth technique is so simple. After removing the meat to use for meals, place everything but the meat back into a crock pot and cover with water a couple of inches over the bones. Cook on low for 15-20 hours. Strain the broth through a colander and discard the bones.

A friend visited me one time when I had some bones cooking in the crock pot. She said my house smelled so good and wanted to know what I was cooking. I told her I was making broth from bones and she exclaimed, "You are such a pioneer!" It's not hard, it's simply forgotten knowledge. Make broth, feed your body!

I don't just drink this broth–I might have a hard time doing that. I use it in soups during the week. Some of our favorites: miso soup, egg drop soup, chicken noodle soup, homemade ramen soup. Your family will love the tasty broth and their bodies will love all the nutrients.

While Westin Price didn't have an alternative to making Bone Broth, you do. There are powdered and pill forms of bone broth that you can purchase and add to your diet every day. There really isn't a good excuse anymore to miss out on this source of valuable vitamins!

Butter and cod liver oil heals cavities

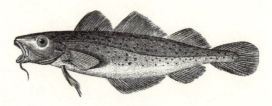

I needed an additional source of these vitamins, so I started taking *Green Pastures Fermented Cod Liver Oil*. I told my team members about it, and they asked me if I was making it myself! I asked them where in the world they thought I would find enough cod to use their livers and extract the oil, then ferment it. I make a lot of things myself, but this isn't one of them!

A good source: www.codliveroilshop.com

½- 1 ½ t per day for adults or in capsule form

Commercial butter that has been pasteurized also contains Vitamin K if it is from grass-fed cows. The store brand I recommend is *KerryGold*, which can be found at most grocery stores. When I told my family we were going to start eating more butter, they cheered, "you finally found a health food we love!!"

I have yet to find someone that doesn't like adding more butter to their diet, but people often wonder how and where to add it. Use it as an added fat at the end of making a dish. Everything tastes amazing with a dollop of butter on it. Every morning we make a *Bulletproof Chocolate Drink* with butter in it. My husband and I do a version of Intermittent Fasting and this is our morning drink.

Good For Your Body Chocolate Drink

3 scoops of ground cocoa beans (the brand we use is *Crio Bru*)
Put into a French Press Coffee Press and cover with boiling water. Let sit for 10 minutes, then press the beans to the bottom and pour the liquid out the top.
Put into a blender with
  6 T butter
  3 T MCT oil
  2 t vanilla
  1 t Truvia sweetener (optional–only my daughter likes this in her drink)

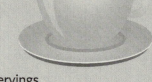

Blend until mixed and drink hot. Makes 3 servings.

The Sugar Dilemma

One key to Dr. Price's research was his use of photographs. He has photo after photo showing the devastating effects of sugar in the diet. But he found it was not always for the reason you think. Remember the "bacteria eats sugar = acid" discussion earlier? It's true that this can lead to cavities, however sugar causes more havoc than just tooth decay.

When we eat sugar, it causes our blood sugar to fluctuate. More sugar in equals more sugar our body must deal with. Did you know that these fluctuating sugar levels affect your bones and teeth? The countries that have the highest sugar consumption rates also have the highest rates of osteoporosis![32]

When you eat more sugar than your body is able to handle all at once, your blood sugars increase. These sugars aren't completely oxidized when they aren't used, and it leads to your body becoming more acidic. When you become acidic, your body automatically reacts by pulling calcium from your bones and teeth to buffer your acidic blood.

The longer your blood sugar is out of balance, the more prone you are to get cavities. White sugar causes the blood sugar to be out of balance for up to five hours, fruit for 4-5 hours and honey for three hours.[1] Bottom line is that eating sugar CAN lead to cavities because of what it does to the BODY and to the TEETH.[33]

One thing I am known for is being a realist. If I tell you never to eat sugar, in any form, you are probably going to give up. What good does that do? Instead I'm going to give you some guidelines and alternatives so you can have your cake (at least a little) and eat it too!

- Take lengthy breaks between eating sweets. If you can give your body time to balance your blood sugar, you can mitigate the effects of the sugar on your teeth. This also gives time for the saliva in your mouth to balance the pH and remineralize areas that have been demineralized. The worst thing you can do is eat small amounts of sugar all day long. I know it feels right to sip one can of soda or nurse one bag of candy all day, but DON'T do it if you want to be healthy!

- Fruit is best with fats (raw cheese, almond butter). The fat fills you up and helps you eat fewer sweets.[34]

- There are "natural" sugars that you should use in place of white sugar. All of them have pros and cons, but here is a short description of why you should use each:

1. Honey

- You can use a smaller amount of honey without sacrificing sweetness.
- It contains traces of vitamins and minerals.
- Raw honey may help alleviate your allergies.

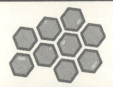

2. Pure Maple Syrup

- Contains antioxidants
- Supplies some vitamins and minerals
- Is anti-inflammatory
- Affects the blood sugar less than white sugar

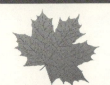

3. Coconut Sugar

- Contains Inulin for gut health – used as a prebiotic to feed good gut bacteria
- Contains vitamins and minerals
- Contains phytonutrients which help reduce blood sugar, inflammation and cholesterol

4. Stevia- make sure you use green leaf stevia or stevia extracts

- Lowers blood pressure
- Improves cholesterol
- Lowers blood sugar

What about Grains and Legumes?

Giving up "carbs," including grains and legumes, is very popular right now. "Keto" and "Paleo" diets are everywhere. What is all this about, and what does it have to do with your teeth?

Because I am a gardener, I am grateful that seeds have a coating on the outside that prevents them from sprouting. I can take a grain of wheat, plant it in the ground, water it, and it will grow. The water washes away the sprouting-inhibitor (called phytic acid) and allows the seed to germinate. The plant then uses the nutrients stored inside that seed to grow and to feed you.

Before it's washed away, this phytic acid holds tightly to the phosphorus in grain, making it unavailable for the seed and the human body to use. It also has "arms" that reach out to bind with calcium, magnesium, iron and zinc. As long as the phytic acid is still coating the grain, the nutrients in the grain are not available for you.

Phosphorus and calcium are the two minerals most essential to tooth remineralization. Dr. Price found that in societies that removed or inactivated this phytic acid before consuming the grain, grains were very nourishing for teeth. On the other hand, if they were not handled correctly, the grains were destructive to the teeth.

Why is it so important to remove/reduce phytic acid (phytates)?

Phytic acid not only grabs on to, or chelates, important minerals, it also also inhibits enzymes that we need to digest our food. These include pepsin needed for the breakdown of proteins in the stomach, amylase needed for the breakdown of starch into sugar, and trypsin needed for protein digestion in the small intestine.[35]

The presence of phytic acid in so many of the foods we are told are "healthy" for us–seeds, nuts and whole grain–makes it crucial that we know how to prepare these foods. The phytic acid needs to be neutralized as much as possible, and these foods should be eaten in a complete diet that helps to counteract the effects of phytic acid.

The ultimate irony is that white rice and white bread are low-phytate foods because their bran and germ have been removed. Yes, they also have very few vitamins and minerals, but the low phytates make them less destructive than their whole grain counterparts that haven't been treated properly.

This may explain why someone whose family eats white flour or white rice food products may seem to be relatively healthy and immune to tooth cavities while those eating whole wheat bread and brown rice could suffer from cavities, bone loss and other health problems. This isn't a "fad." Handling grains, nuts and seeds properly is essential to health.

Consumption of high levels of phytic acid leads to:

1. mineral deficiencies, leading to poor bone health and tooth decay
2. blocked absorption of zinc, iron, phosphorous and magnesium
3. leeching of calcium from the body
4. lowered metabolism
5. anemia

Make the nutrients in grains available for your body

People living in traditional cultures throughout the world had lives filled with time-consuming daily activities. Yet they soaked, fermented, and ground their grains before using them. They often removed the hull of the grain before use as well. Why did they take the time? Because they knew it was the only way to get all the nutrients out of the grain. [36,37]

Aren't we more advanced than these societies? Don't we have science and research on our side? Unfortunately, in today's "ready-made" world, nearly all grains and legumes aren't handled in these traditional ways. Our world demands fast, and these traditional methods are not fast.

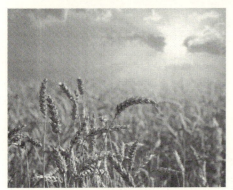

Grains and legumes can be very hard to absorb and digest, especially modern-day grains. While agricultural societies have been living for thousands of years on grains, the grains we use have been hybridized and changed in the last 50+ years, and our handling of them has been significantly altered.

The amount of phytate in grains, nuts, legumes and seeds varies greatly based on growing conditions, harvesting techniques, processing methods and even the age of the food being tested. Phytic acid will be much higher in foods grown using modern high-phosphate fertilizers than those grown in natural compost.[38]

Remember the oat bran fad of the 1980s? Eating bran, or high fiber foods containing different types of bran will lead directly to bone loss and digestive problems due to the high phytic acid content. We have forgotten how to make these foods good for our bodies.

This change in the way grains and legumes are grown and handled before eating has led, in part, to the exponential rise in gluten intolerance and other digestive problems that run rampant today, like leaky gut.

What are these traditional ways of handling grains and legumes?

Phytase to the Rescue! Phytase is a natural enzyme present in varying amounts inside of grains, seeds and nuts. When this enzyme is activated, it works to break down the phytic acid, and helps to release the nutrients that are so crucial for healthy teeth. It also makes the grain, nut or seed more digestible.

Unfortunately, cooking is not enough to adequately release phytase and reduce phytic acid. You must pre-treat the grains, seeds and nuts in one of two ways: [39-47]

- Soaking grains/flour in an acid medium at a warm temperature–helps to reduce, or even eliminate phytic acid.[48]
- Souring—think sourdough bread with natural yeast. This is the preferred method for reducing phytic acid in breads and bread-products.

In general, the best means of significantly reducing phytic acid in grains and legumes is a combination of acidic soaking for a long time, followed by cooking.

One important thing to note is that not all grains contain enough phytase to eliminate the phytic acid, even when they are soaked. Oats and corn are two of these. So when soaking, if you add a small amount of a high phytase flour (rye, wheat, spelt and kamut) to the soaking water for corn and oats, it will help reduce the high phytase in these two grains

Bottom line...If you want to eat grains and/or legumes, you must soak or ferment them before eating!

How to Soak

On any given night, you may find random bowls and measuring cups littering my countertop. These hold grains, nuts, seeds and legumes that are soaking before I use them for meals later in the week. Soaking isn't hard, in fact, it's really easy. The hard part is that you have to plan ahead, which is difficult in today's fast paced world. This is not "fast food", but it's good for your body food, so I believe it's worth it.

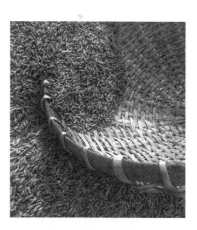

Here is what you need to soak grains, seeds, nuts, flour & legumes:

- Filtered water ~ warm water is necessary to properly break down the phytic acid and other minerals.
- Some kind of acid - yogurt*, buttermilk*, lemon juice, apple cider vinegar, whey, milk kefir* and coconut kefir. *If using dairy it needs to be cultured.
- Baking soda for legumes
- Time

Soaking Grains, Nuts and Seeds[50]

Put grain into a glass bowl and cover completely with filtered water. **For every 1 cup of liquid you will need 1 tbsp of acid.** (Most grains: soak for 12-24 hours. Buckwheat, brown rice and millet: soak for 7 hours).

1. Cover bowl
2. Rinse in a colander after soaking.
3. Use in the recipe (may take less time to cook after they are soaked)
4. You can grind these grains wet in a Food Processor

Michelle's Living Granola

- 4 c almonds
- 1 c pecan pieces
- 1 c walnuts
- 1 c pumpkin seeds
- 1 c sunflower seeds
- 2 c raisins
- 2 T vanilla extract
- 1 t cinnamon
- 1 t salt
- ½ c hemp seeds
- ½ c flax seeds
- 2 c oats
- ½ c shredded, unsweetened coconut
- 1 c raisins
- 1 c craisins or apricots

1. Place nuts and seeds in a large bowl, cover with water and soak 12 hours.
2. Place raisins in a small bowl with 1-2 C water to cover and soak 12 hours.
3. Place raisins, along with their soaking water in food processor and puree until smooth
4. Drain and rinse nuts and seeds and discard soaking water.
5. Add to raisin puree in the food processor and pulse until coarsely chopped (may have to do this in two batches – if so use half the raisin puree in each batch)
6. Add vanilla, cinnamon, salt, hemp seed, flax seed and oats and pulse until mixed.
7. Mix both batches together and spread onto Teflex sheets in dehydrator sheets or onto baking sheets for the oven.
8. Dehydrate for 12-24 hours until dry all the way through. If using the oven, leave on the "warm" setting or turn oven on as low as it will go and cook until dry, 8-12 hours.
9. Place in large bowl and add coconut, raisins and craisins. Mix and break granola pieces up to desired size.
10. Store granola in the refrigerator.

Soaking flours

If soaking flour, you start making the recipe the night before, adding the flours and the water, oil and sweetener. Mix in a glass bowl and cover overnight.

Add the other ingredients in the morning and continue making the recipe (eggs, milk, etc). Remember this includes nut flours, like almond flour, that are high in phytic acid as well.

Overnight Sourdough Pancake Recipe

1 c sourdough starter
2 c water
2 ½ c flour (whole wheat or white)
1 T sugar or honey

1 egg
2 T olive oil
½ t salt
1 t baking soda

In a large glass bowl or measuring cup, mix the sourdough starter, water, flour and sweetener. Cover and leave overnight. In the morning add the egg, olive oil and salt. Stir until mixed. If it is very thick add 1-2 T water to thin.

Mix the baking soda in 1 T water and add to the pancake mix. Will bubble up. Cook the pancakes on a hot griddle. Makes about 16 pancakes.

Soaking legumes

1. For kidney shaped beans, add enough water to cover the beans and a pinch of baking soda. Cover and allow to sit in a warm kitchen for 12-24 hours, changing the water and baking soda once or twice.

2. For non kidney shaped beans such as northern beans or black beans, place beans into pot and add enough "hot to the touch" water to cover the beans. For every one cup of beans you can add 1 tbsp of acid like vinegar or lemon juice, however it does slightly change the flavor and texture of the cooked bean. Soak for 12-24 hours and change the soaking water at least once.

3. After soaking is done, rinse the beans, replace the water and cook for 4-8 hours on low heat or for 6-8 hour on high in the crockpot until beans are tender.

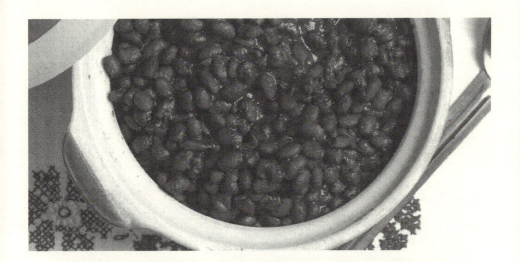

All-Day Crockpot Black Beans

Place **2 cups of beans** in a crockpot and cover with water. Add **2 T apple cider vinegar**. Soak overnight or 12-24 hours. Change water and vinegar at least once if soaking longer than overnight. Rinse the beans in clean water, then cover again with water, adding enough to have one inch of water above the level of the beans.

Optional: Add **1 t epazote** (a spice found in Hispanic markets) or **1 piece kombu seaweed** (found dried in Asian markets) for flavor and to help decrease gas after eating.

Cook in your crockpot on high for 6-7 hours. Add water if needed during cooking time if the beans absorb all of the water. When soft, mash them as much as desired in the crock pot and add salt to taste.

Rice—Use partially milled white rice or brown rice that has been soaked overnight and up to 24 hours. Drain and rinse rice, then cook as normal.

All societies that use rice as a staple food eat white rice. It's more work to create white rice, so why do they go to the effort? Because they learned through centuries that their bodies felt better if they removed the hull before eating the rice. The phytic acid and other plant lectins (inflammatory proteins the plant uses for defense) are in the hull of the rice.

On the other hand, there are more nutrients available in brown rice. To get the best of both worlds, presoak the brown rice for digestibility and increased nutrition.

> **Simple Soaked Brown Rice**
>
> *1 cup of organic brown rice*
> *1T raw apple cider vinegar or lemon juice*
> *2 cup warm filtered water*
> *⅛ t salt*
>
> Add ingredients to a glass bowl and thoroughly combine. Cover the bowl and leave overnight in warm area in kitchen. Drain over a fine strainer and rinse well.
>
> Put drained rice in a pan and add 1¾ cup of water or bone broth. Bring to a boil then cover and reduce heat until it is gently simmering. Cook 25-40 minutes until rice has absorbed the liquid and reached the consistency you desire.

Corn—There are two big problems with corn today. These problems impact us because corn is often used as a filler in processed foods. First, there is very little corn that is not GMO today. GMO stands for "Genetically Modified Organisms". This corn is modified to grow faster, to be resistant to weeds and insects, to have more efficient processing, but not to be healthier for us. Second, very often corn is not treated correctly, which can lead to malnutrition and a disease called pellagra.

Maize, or corn, has been a staple food in central America for thousands of years, with indigenous peoples soaking the dried corn kernels in alkaline lye or quicklime before cooking. This is called "nixtamalization," and it increases the bioavailability of bound niacin (Vitamin B3) in the corn by converting it into a water-soluble free compound, allowing it to be absorbed by the gut.

Because of this traditional preparation method, the native people of the Americas did not suffer from nutritional disease like pellagra. These diseases came later when traditional food handling methods were discarded.

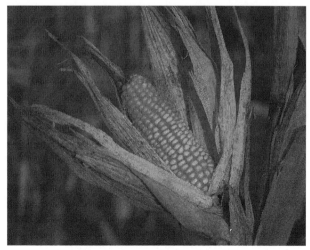

The Corn Tragedy

Maize or corn was unknown to the European settlers when they arrived in the Americas, but they saw it as a lifeline. It was low in cost and it provided high yields. The indigenous people showed the settlers how to prepare the corn before turning it into a dough by first soaking it in lime water (North American Indians used wood ash water), then rinsing the corn before grinding it into corn mash. This process came to be known as *Nixtamalization*. However, for the Europeans, the process was time consuming, and it seemed unnecessary. What good did it do? They thought it was probably just another superstition of these uncivilized people.

What happened next is an untold tragedy in history. Corn became a staple in the diet for many people in parts of Europe, Africa, India, and China, but without nixtamalization. The result was thousands of people dying from a disease called pellagra, caused by a chronic lack of niacin (Vitamin B3) in the diet.

Here in the Americas the tragedy continued when these traditional practices were not handed down. In the Southern states, in the economic downturn following the American Civil War, the diet for poor people consisted almost entirely of corn-based products such as cornbread and grits. The devastation occurred on a grand scale; across the United States from 1906 to 1940 approximately 3 million cases and 100,000 deaths were attributed to pellagra.

Not until 1938 was the link between niacin deficiency and pellagra widely understood. But long before that time, the link between a staple diet of corn and pellagra had been noticed. It was believed that eating corn somehow caused the disease, possibly through insects, or a toxin, or a disease which lived on the corn. But the true culprit was a diet in which corn was the exclusive grain, and not treated properly before consuming.[51-57]

How to Make Lime Water [58]

Filtered water
Pickling Lime or Cal Mexicana (calcium hydroxide) (Can be found in the canning section of a store, in a Hispanic Market, or online.)

Place about a ½ cup of the pickling lime into a 1 quart Mason jar. Fill the jar with water, screw on the lid and shake. Let the jar stand on the counter for a few hours until the lime settles, leaving you with a mildly cloudy liquid.

Use the cloudy liquid at the top as your lime water. Save the rest for use later – it does not go bad when stored at room temperature.

Soaking Corn

2 cups dried organic, non-GMO corn (Great River Organic Milling)
1 T pickling lime
8 cups water

Rinse the corn, then add to a non-reactive pan (stainless steel or ceramic). Cover with the water and add the lime. Bring to a boil then reduce to a simmer for 30 minutes. Remove from the heat and allow to sit for 6-16 hours or overnight.

After the soaking, rinse in water with a strainer and rub the kernels between your fingers to remove some of the skins (don't have to remove them all).

Making Tortillas

Place rinsed corn into a food processor. Add half of the corn, with ½ t salt and ¼ C water and grind until a smooth dough forms. Repeat with the other half of the corn. Can add a small amount of masa harina if it's too wet. Refrigerate for 1-2 hours. Form into balls and flatten with a tortilla press. Cook in a hot pan or griddle.

If using cornmeal

If soaking cornmeal, use 1 cup of the lime water for every 2 cups of cornmeal. Allow the mixture to stand at room temperature for 12 hours then proceed as needed for your desired recipe.

Oats

Oats are the exception to the soaking rule. In Dr. Westin Price's research, he found that the societies that consumed a lot of oats had a significant increase in tooth decay. This didn't make sense to me, so I continued researching until I found out why.

Oats contain a large amount of hard-to-digest phytates and other anti-nutrients. And I also learned that oats are so low in phytase, the enzyme that helps to break down phytates, that soaking them as described above is not enough to break down naturally occurring antinutrients. But there is a trick that can make them safe to use.

> **Soaking Oats**
>
> 1 cup oat groats or flakes
> Warm filtered water to cover the oats
> 1 T apple cider vinegar or lemon juice
> 1 T spelt or wheat flour, rye flour or rolled rye flakes -or- ground buckwheat groats for a gluten-free version
>
> Soak for a full 24 hours, drain and rinse in a fine mesh strainer and cook as usual.

What if You Are Eating Correctly and Still Not Getting the Nutrients You Need?

Let's go back to the story at the beginning of this chapter about the nutrition and health author with multiple cavities. I have patients that come every day with similar stories. They are doing most of the things in this chapter right. They are handling their food properly, they are getting the food from good sources, they are avoiding sugar and other processed foods, yet they *still* have cavities and other dental issues. This is when we start looking at digestive function and the way the gut is working.

If the stomach and digestive functions are not working properly, you can eat the most wonderful food in the world and it won't do you as much good as it should. Often the problem is lack of stomach acid and it's because we are all living in a stressful world. When you are experiencing stress, including mental stress, physical stress from dental, food, and medical issues or environmental stress like wifi and cell frequencies around us, your body doesn't create enough stomach acid to digest foods.

This stomach acid, called hydrochloric acid, is essential for three things.
1. Proper digestion of proteins
2. Proper digestion of minerals
3. Protection from harmful microbes.

I find that many people are deficient in this essential stomach acid, which can lead to many problems other than heartburn.

Low stomach acid, called hypochlorhydria, can cause gas, bloating, diarrhea, malabsorption of nutrients, iron-deficiency anemia, dry and thin skin and hair, acne, dysbiosis (improper balance of gut bacteria), allergies, chronic fatigue, a weakened immune system and can aggravate arthritis and other inflammatory conditions.

How do you know if this is your problem? Here is an easy health test you can do at home to confirm or rule this out.

Baking soda test to determine stomach acid level

Carry out the following steps to determine your stomach's acidity.

1. Perform this test first thing in the morning on an empty stomach (before eating or drinking).
2. Dissolve ¼ teaspoon of baking soda into an 8 oz. glass of cold water.
3. Drink the solution and start timing.
4. Record the time until you first burp up gas.
5. Perform this test for four consecutive days (or longer) at the same time each day to give a better estimation of your stomach's acidity.

Day	Time Until First Burp
1	
2	
3	
4	

Interpreting your results:
- 2 minutes: indicates normal acidity
- 2-3 minutes: indicates low-normal acidity
- 3 minutes: possible hypochlorhydria

If you find that your stomach acid levels are low, you need to work with a holistic health practitioner to do two things.
1. You need to supplement with HCL acid to digest now. Can add digestive enzymes and probiotics to help.
2. You need to determine the cause of the low acid and build it up with things like iodine, zinc and B vitamins.

Chapter Six: Clean Up Past Problems

There are some long-standing controversies in dentistry. These controversies are like land-mines that traditional dentistry has to tread carefully around. In our litigious society, if it were discovered that any dental practices were harmful, every dentist in the country would be included in a massive class-action law suit. In order to avoid this, the large dental associations have taken very "safe" stances in regard to the topics we will discuss in this chapter. Fortunately, there are very logical, science-based explanations of the dangers and realities of these treatments. I'm going to share the "in the trenches" reasons why you should or shouldn't have these procedures done and let you make your own decisions about what is best for you.

What is a Root Canal?

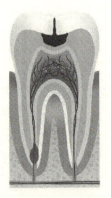
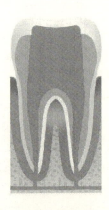
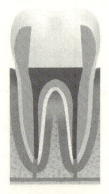

Infected Tooth   **Tooth Cleaned And Shaped**   **Root Filling And Crown Replaced**

This is where your new found knowledge of tooth anatomy will come in handy. A better name for the procedure is a "root filled tooth". The nerve inside a tooth can get inflamed or infected from a very large cavity, or from trauma. Remember that this nerve is inside the center of each tooth. If the inflammation or infection leads to the nerve dying, there are only two options for the tooth at this time (new stem cell therapies are being developed but are not ready for clinical use).

Option #1 – pull the tooth.

Option #2 – Remove the nerve tissue in the center of the tooth and down the root, and fill the area with a material called gutta percha (a rubber-like material from Malaysian trees).

In the 1800s when modern dentistry was in its infancy, dentists and their patients were frustrated because so many teeth had to be pulled. They experimented with removing the infected and dead nerve tissue, rinsing and disinfecting the inside of the tooth, and filling it. The techniques and materials have evolved, and today more that 22 million root canals are performed every year in the US alone.[1] Why? To "save" teeth that have been neglected or damaged. The tooth is no longer alive, but it is retained in the jaw bone to continue functioning.

The problem with root canals

Dentists are usually quite successful in cleaning out the main root canal area and disinfecting it. In fact, in most cases, even the infected bone at the end of the root will heal and new bone grows in it's place after the procedure. If so, what is the problem?

Let's go back to that anatomy lesson. Remember that dentin is made up of miles of tubules, all filled with a lymph-like fluid. Each of those tubules opens into the center nerve chamber in the tooth. The bacteria that are involved in tooth decay travel through those dentin tubules to get from the outside to the inside of the tooth in order to infect the nerve. Think of it as the highway system of the tooth.

The medications used to sterilize a tooth are very effective at cleaning the main root canal area, but not the tubules. There are simply too many of them. Once the root is filled, the fluid that fills those tubules and the bacteria they contain back up like a plugged sewer. The tubules are a nice place for the bacteria to hide, and your immune system or any antibiotic can't get to them because the flushing system in the tooth has been removed.

Those trapped bacteria have to adapt to living with no oxygen, and these new "anaerobic" *(without oxygen)* bacteria create waste products called endotoxins. Those toxins are the thing that cause harm as they freely circulate in the bloodstream and around the end of the tooth.

This causes the bone around the tooth to become very unhealthy. The nerve is gone so the tooth often doesn't hurt, but those endotoxins are affecting your jawbone and your body. This low-grade infection causes your immune system to stand guard constantly. Eventually, your immune system wears out from working overtime, and when there is an invader somewhere else in the body, it won't have enough fresh troops to send to fight. Sickness, fatigue, chronic illness and autoimmune disease are all conditions that can come because of an overtaxed immune system. And that reinfected root canal tooth can contribute to the overtaxing.

Why Dentists Don't Know This

I used to be out on a limb when talking about the problems with root canals, but recent research has supported and validated these concerns many times over. In a comprehensive research article published in the Jan-Mar 2016 *European Journal of Dentistry*[2], the problems and potential pitfalls of root canals were explained very clearly. Interestingly, none of these are new to dentists.

Any dental student or dentist can tell you where a root canal can go wrong and is taught how to avoid the problems. However, there are so many potential areas of failure, it is difficult to perform a "perfect" root canal.[3]

As the article explains, the "usual suspects" are:

- Bacteria remaining in the root[4]
- Leaking of the root canal filling material[5]
- The filling material ending up too short or too long for the root[6]
- Leaking fillings or crowns on top of the root canal tooth[7]
- Instruments breaking inside the root during the procedure[8]
- Completely missing one or more of the canals when cleaning out the root[9]

Whew... that's a lot of things to do perfectly every time, reducing the chance that every root canal will be perfect. The odds are stacked against long term success with root canals, and indeed, studies are showing that failures do occur at some point in the life span of the root-filled teeth.[10]

Research About Root Canals

The first research was done more than 100 years ago by Dr. Westin Price. He was the head of research for the *National Dental Association*, the precursor to the current *American Dental Association*. He tried to sterilize teeth with the chemicals that are used today in root canal treatments. He found that out of 1,000 "sterilized," extracted teeth, he could culture dangerous bacteria out of 990 of them after only two days.[11]

Don't just take my word for this. Dr. Josef Issels, MD, a world-famous cancer specialist, was one of the first doctors to require all of his cancer patients to have their root-canaled teeth removed as part of his healing protocol. In his book, Cancer: A Second Opinion, he explains that during 40 years of working with 16,000 thousand cancer patients, over 90% of his patients had between two and ten root-canaled teeth in their mouths. He believes that root-canaled teeth generate toxins that can lead to cancer. Dr. Jerry Tennant, in his book Healing is Voltage: Cancer's On/Off Switches, stated that he finds 90% of cancers are related to a diseased tooth.

In a 2013 study[12] published by Dr. Tanja Pessi and others in the American Heart Association's journal, Circulation, they show that failed root canals play a significant role in heart attacks and strokes. In a study of the clots and blood samples from 101 people that had had a fatal heart attack, it was discovered that 78.2% of the clots had oral bacteria that cause root canal abscesses and 34.7% of the clots contained bacteria found in periodontal disease. X-rays from 30 of the patients found that 50% had infected teeth. These research findings suggest that up to 50% of heart attacks may be triggered by an infection in the mouth.

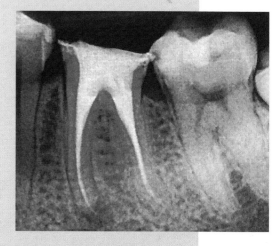

This research study was ground breaking in many ways, and follow-up research has affirmed what the study found. See a list of follow-up studies in the list of sources at the end of the book.[13-17]

Should a Root Canaled Tooth be Removed?

This is where it gets sticky. Traditional dentists will usually recommend a root canal for infected or dead teeth, and a redo or surgical root canal (called an apicoectomy) if that root canal fails. In fact, I myself have performed hundreds of root canals in my career, but I no longer offer or perform the procedure. Why the change?

I now use a specialized dental xray called a Cone Beam CT scan that shows the teeth and surrounding bone in 3D. I can see teeth and root canals and the bone surrounding the root canals in a way I never could before–and every day I see failed root canals. In fact, nearly every new patient that I visit with has at least one failed root canal. I see so much infection and disease I can no longer offer that procedure myself. I still tell my patients about the root canal option, as I am required to do by law, but I refer them to a root canal specialist (endodontist) if they choose to have a root canal.

Does this mean there is no other choice than to remove a tooth that is dead or dying? Some of the most convincing research completed in this area was again by our friend Dr. Weston Price. In his day, root canal filling and sealing materials were much less successful than they are today, so you might think he would make this "pull every infected tooth" recommendation. He didn't.[11]

There are people that have had root canal treatments completed years ago, and the tooth has not reinfected, and they have remained in good health. Dr. Price found that this was about 30% of those treated. He said, "I am not ready to draw the line so rigidly to state that all root-filled teeth should be extracted for every patient or for all patients in any given time, though I do believe there is a limit of safety for all such teeth for each and every patient."

Can You Have a Successful Root Canal?

What is the key to a successful root canal? The health of the person getting the root canal! People with strong immune systems and no family tendency to chronic degenerative disease can possibly have and retain successful root canal fillings.

Here's the catch twenty-two. Dr. Price found that if those healthy people had an accident, caught a flu-bug, had a death in the family, or suffered some other severe stress, their immune system became over stressed. When the immune system is over stressed, it must drop the ball on a few things, and those trapped bacteria may multiply and start causing problems. A healthy person with a root canal may not stay healthy. This means a non-problematic root canal may become a problem–even years in the future.

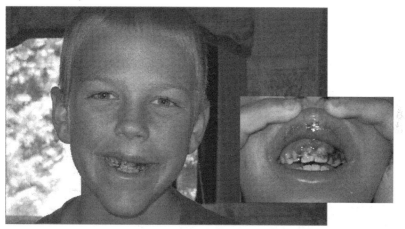

What to do, what to do?! I was faced with this very personal situation a few years ago with my 11 year old son. While warming up for an All-Stars baseball game, he got hit in the mouth with a baseball. He came around the corner spitting out teeth, and my heart just sank. I knew what he was in for. One of his front teeth came out and was not savable, and the other front tooth was fractured ½ way down the root but didn't come out. My choice was to do a root canal to save the tooth for now, or take out both of my son's permanent front teeth. It makes me sick to my stomach to think about it even years later!

I chose to do a root canal. And in his situation, with a fractured root, I 100% know his root canal will leak and fail. Why did I make this choice? He was very healthy, in the middle of a big growth spurt, and I could keep an eye on his health and the tooth. His body should be able to handle the root canal for a few years until he has grown enough to permanently replace the tooth.

I view root canals as temporary solutions. They help retain the tooth in the mouth, keep the space and buy time for the patient to stop growing or find a better solution.

Recommendations

There is not a hard-and-fast answer to the root canal controversy. I can't give you a rule, but from what I've observed with hundreds of patients, I've come up with some recommendations.

- If you are in that 30% category of healthy immune system and no family history of degenerative disease like diabetes, arthritis, heart disease or cancer, you have a statistically higher chance for a successful root canal right now. You may get 5, 10, even 15 years more with that tooth.

- If you are in the 70% category with some immune problems, any existing degenerative diseases (arthritis, heart problems, diabetes, etc) or a family history of degenerative diseases, you have a statistically lower chance for a successful root canal. You may wish to extract the tooth rather than pay for a root canal and have it fail and negatively affect your health.

- If you have an existing root canal and have have nagging, unexplained medical problems, or progressive degenerative diseases or immune problems, your root canal may be contributing to your health problems.

- If you have an existing root canal and are in good health, AND if the tooth appears healthy and uninfected on a diagnostic xray (CT scan is the only method to view this), you may choose to leave the tooth there for now.

Warning: Any good holistic dentist will let you know that removal of a root canal tooth may not fully alleviate the illness you feel may be related to that tooth. There are often multiple "foundational problems" that contribute to your illness or disease, the root canal being one. If enough of these foundational problems are removed, the body is able to heal. Improving nutrition, correcting stomach acid, and rebuilding your energy systems are all important pieces your holistic dentist should be able to help with as well.

The best root canal is no root canal at all. Except in trauma situations like my son's, most root canals can be avoided with proper care and nutrition. Please read the chapters on *Tooth Care and Diet* again. You don't ever want to have to make the difficult decision to keep or remove a tooth. If you do have a very deep cavity, make sure to read the section on *Biomimetic and Tooth Preserving Dentistry* before getting a root canal. There are treatment options, including ozone, that can be used to seal and heal a tooth that may otherwise have required a root canal.

Twenty First Century Dental Options

There are new advances in all areas of dentistry, including root canals. Some things are in the experimental stages, while others are being used by a few pioneering dentists. Things to watch for:

- **Laser sterilization of root canal areas–** There is hope that use of a laser during the root canal procedure can sterilize the root area and keep bacteria out. To date this has not prevented regrowth of these damaging bacteria, but the technology is advancing every day.

- **Ozone sterilization of root canal areas**[18]**–** Ozone is a very powerful anti-microbial. One molecule of ozone is more powerful than 3000 molecules of bleach (which is standard of care for disinfecting root canals right now). But ozone is a gas, and it leaves the area quickly. The root canal is completely disinfected at the time it's filled, but the effect of the ozone does not last and the bacteria regrow. Ozone research is at the leading edge of medical and dental innovation, so I will be anxiously watching for solutions to this problem.

- **Antimicrobial root filling materials–** This is up and coming technology. There are also experiments using root canal sealing materials made of ceramics, in hopes the root canal will not leak. This would prevent leakage, but leakage isn't the only problem. The bacteria congregate at the end of the root canal, outside of the root, as well. Nothing has been shown to inhibit growth there yet.

- **Oral probiotics**[19]**–** These are specialized beneficial oral bacteria. The thought is, if the destructive bacteria are overpowered by beneficial mouth bacteria, there is less likelihood the tooth will re-infect. Again, the problem is that unless you continually take these probiotics, the effect does not last.

- **Helping a tooth regrow the nerve–** This is the one I'm most excited about! Bodies are able to heal in so many other ways, there must be a way to help teeth heal as well. I will be one of the first to adopt this treatment, if and when it becomes clinically viable.

What can you do if you already have a root canal tooth?

Option #1 – Have it removed. No one likes this option. People don't like going without teeth, or paying to have them replaced, and dentists don't like removing them! Root canal teeth have lost the ligament surrounding them and they are often "cemented" to the bone, making these teeth difficult to remove.

Despite this difficulty, I am recommending and removing teeth on a greater number of patients than ever before. I used to recommend saving a tooth at any cost, and now I save health at any cost, even if it means losing a tooth. Keep that in mind when making your decision.

Option #2 – Keep it healthy. How can you keep a dead tooth healthy? You can help the health of the tooth by keeping your body healthy.

There are two additional dental procedures you can choose from to prolong the life of the root canal tooth.

> *I used to recommend saving a tooth at any cost, and now I save health at any cost, even if it means losing a tooth.*

1. Non-metal crown. This one is a little mad-scientist like. If you have a metal filling or crown or porcelain crown with a metal core, you have a small battery in your mouth (You can't always see the metal core, and can check to see if there is one with a dental xray). All fillings and metal containing crowns are made out of an alloy, which is a combination of different metals. In saliva, those metals have a small electrical current running between them. You may have felt like "you are chewing on tin foil". That's the current I'm talking about. It's called galvanism.[20]

Bacteria love this small current and they flourish when it's there. If you have a metal filling or crown on the tooth with a root canal, you've created the perfect storm. The metals are attracting bacteria and the bacteria are re-infecting the root canal. Solution–have the metal replaced with porcelain.

2. Good bugs. We all have millions of microbes in our mouths. Some are good and some are bad. If you have a root canal that you would like to keep healthy, give your mouth an extra boost by taking a special probiotic formulated for mouths. There are many brands available online now, including *Florassist* by *Life Extension*, a lozenge shown through research to reduce infection in the mouth.

Interesting to note – just like you can pass on those flu bugs, you can pass on your cavity bugs too. If you and your mom have bad teeth, it's probably as much about mom giving you her bad bugs as it is about genetics. A probiotic can turn this around for you and your family.

IMPORTANT: Root Canal Tooth Removal Protocol

There is a very specific protocol that must be followed when removing the root canal tooth in order the ensure the bone heals properly.

Remember the ligament that surrounds the root of the tooth? It's called the periodontal ligament. If your tooth is infected, this ligament is infected as well. After the tooth is removed, the ligament and a thin layer of bone surrounding the tooth must be removed.

If this infected area isn't removed, the body takes 14 days to realize the tooth is gone. During that time the body has started to heal over the top, "capping" a hole in the bone rather than filling the hole in. This hole could be a source of long standing bone infection and toxins. The action of removing this ligament and the surrounding thin layer of bone also turns on the cells that help the bone in the area regenerate. This is a simple step you can ask a dentist to perform to help any tooth removal area heal.

Jaw Bone Infection and Bony Cavitations.

If the area where a tooth is removed doesn't heal properly, a hole persists in the bone. A hole is called a cavity, so these jaw bones holes have been called cavitations. These holes contain dead or dying bone and microbial infections.[22]

The first jaw bone cavitations were found in the early 1900s and were called NICO lesions (Neuralgia Inducing Cavitational Osteonecrosis) . Further research by German toxicologists has shown these jaw bone holes to contain a slew of chemicals and heavy metals.

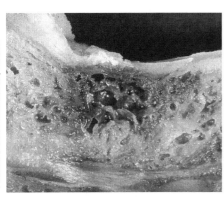
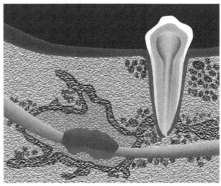

Photo: J Oral Pathol Med 1999; 28:423.

These cavitations are found in areas where the teeth have been removed, usually in the wisdom tooth area. I find that a large majority of people have one or more areas where a wisdom tooth has been removed that has an unhealed cavity in the bone.

Why are bony cavitations a problem?

These cavitations block the blood supply to the bone, which leads to further bone death and a larger area of cavitation. These can be found on a dental specific CBCT scan, and I highly recommend you be screened for them by a dentist that is able to read the CT scan and look for areas of decreased bone density.[23-26]

These toxic sinkholes contain microbes that impair your energy production. This can slow you down and lead to fatigue, brain fog and other energy related problems. In fact, cavitations have been linked to Chronic Fatigue Syndrome.[27-30]

There is current research in Germany also showing a correlation between these bone cavitations and other serious systemic diseases such as cancer, autoimmune disease, inflammatory disease, including heart disease and arthritis, and brain and nerve problems.[31-38]

How to treat cavitations

There are few dentists who know how to diagnose bony cavitations properly, and even fewer who know how to treat them. My recommendation is to find a dentist with significant experience removing the dead bone and disinfecting the site, as well as stimulating the area to heal and grow new bone. This is a very specialized surgery that needs to be done with care.

Success Story:

Stacey was sick and didn't know why. She was in her early 30s, and had to quit a career she loved and move back in with her parents. She spent most of her days in bed, waking up late and lacking the energy to even get out of bed. She gained unexplained weight, had chronic energy issues, and her mother was afraid Stacey might not make it through these challenges.

They had been to so many doctors, tried so many things, and nothing had made significant improvement in her health or her energy. She was referred to my office to see if she had bony cavitations. On a

CBCT scan, we found areas areas of cavitated bone in all of her wisdom tooth removal sites. She also had an infected root canal tooth.

In one appointment, all of the cavitation areas were opened up, cleaned, sterilized and a stem cell containing product from her own blood was placed into the areas to encourage growth. The root canal tooth was also removed and an immediate ceramic implant was placed. She reported feeling more like herself the afternoon of the surgery, and the next day her mother found her doing dishes, rather than in bed for the first time in years.

Stacey started walking, and is now walking eight miles each day. She just left on a long-awaited trip to China that she never thought she would be able to take. Cleaning up her past dentistry saved her life.

Mercury Fillings

On to the next controversy! This one also affects a large majority of the population and stirs up a lot of debate. Let's talk about "silver amalgam" fillings.

> *"There is mercury in silver fillings?! They don't put mercury in anymore, do they?"*

The first mercury dental filling material was made in France in 1816. A Frenchman mixed mercury with shavings from silver coins and formed a soft paste that could easily be packed into a hole in the tooth. It took a few minutes to turn hard, so it could be shaped to fit the tooth well. This was brought to the US in 1830 and was an instant success. This new filling material was inexpensive, easy to use, lasted a long time, and sealed the tooth fairly well. It became popular very quickly.

That first filling material was 50% mercury (the liquid shiny stuff in thermometers) and 50% silver. When I told a friend who was a successful professional outside of dentistry about my health problems from mercury, he looked confused. "There is mercury in silver fillings?! They don't put mercury in, anymore, do they?"

I'm afraid so. In fact, 50% of those "silver" fillings today and 150 years ago, are mercury, despite widespread knowledge that mercury is one of the most deadly metals on the planet, known to cause massive, irreversible neurological damage. Mercury can damage not only your brain but all of your nervous system.

The International Academy of Oral Medicine and Toxicology (IAOMT), a dental organization seeking to bring awareness to the public and to change policy for mercury fillings, wrote a position paper in 2016 about

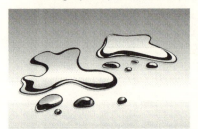

mercury fillings. The organization said, *"Thus, while these restorations are commonly referred to as 'silver fillings,' 'dental amalgam,' and/or 'amalgam fillings,' the public is often unaware that amalgam refers to the combination of other metals with mercury."*

A 2014 Zogby poll established that 57% of Americans did not know that mercury is the main ingredient in amalgam fillings and that 63% thought the commonplace practice of referring to mercury amalgams as "silver fillings" was misleading. It would be more appropriate therefore to recognize them as "dental mercury amalgam fillings," "mercury silver fillings," or "mercury fillings."

If we remove a mercury filling, the EPA tells us we have to treat that piece of filling like a toxic substance, and I had to install new mercury separators on my vacuum lines to make sure none of the mercury enters the water supply. You might ask why it's safe in your mouth and not in the water.[39]

If you break a mercury-containing thermometer, there are nine intense steps you are to take to collect and dispose of the mercury, including calling the fire department to dispose of it. We are warned about eating too much fish because of the mercury in the fish. Mercury toxicity is not a secret or anything anyone will debate with you. So why are dentists still placing these fillings?

Recently, I talked to a dentist who graduated from dental school in 2011. I explained my concerns about my patients and myself breathing in mercury vapors as I remove old mercury fillings. He said he's never heard anything about it. He didn't know it could be a problem for patients or dentists. He graduated in recent years and was taught to place mercury fillings and routinely places them in his practice now. This is not new information. It's obvious the dental community at large doesn't understand the problem.

How mercury fillings began

When this material was introduced, barber/dentists did much of the dental work, and they loved these new fillings. They were easy to place, and they could make money on them. The few doctors that did dentistry at that time were not so excited about it. They knew the symptoms of mercury exposure from watching hat makers. The hat makers would use mercury to turn fur into felt. After repeated exposure to this mercury, the hat makers started showing bizarre behavior. This is where the term "mad hatter" comes from. The mercury quite literally was making them crazy![40]

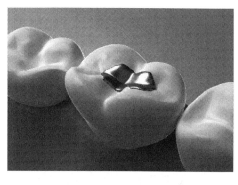

The doctors were concerned that mercury was being placed into teeth, but the barbers continued placing them. They were making money on these easy fillings. Mercury/silver fillings were here to stay.[41]

Toxic material

That is the background behind dental mercury fillings, and they are still being used today in nearly 50% of the dental offices in the US. They are called "silver" fillings or "amalgam" fillings, but the components are all the same. There are quite a few dentists, such as myself and the doctors that work with me, that have abandoned them because the safety and science just doesn't make sense.

I was attending a meeting in Switzerland recently and was one of only two dentists from the US at the course. I overheard a conversation between a dentist from England and a dentist from Australia. They were complaining that their governments only regulated amalgam use in children and pregnant women. I told them it was much worse in the U.S. Dentists here can put mercury amalgam fillings in anyone, at any age. There are no regulations.

> *The EU Regulation states that, from 1 July 2018, dental amalgam should not be used in the treatment of children under 15 years of age and in pregnant or breastfeeding women, except when deemed strictly necessary by the dental practitioner based on the specific medical needs of the patient.*
> https://bda.org/dentists/policy-campaigns/public-health-science/dental-amalgam-faqs

I am often asked why our government or the FDA or the ADA (*American Dental Association*) doesn't place regulations on these mercury fillings. This is a difficult question to answer because it's loaded with legalities and politics. The ADA was sued over this years ago, and stated that they had no duty to the public in regards to amalgam fillings because the dentist "manufactures" the filling at the time of use, so the dentist is the responsible party.[42]

If the FDA changed its classification of mercury fillings, declaring them unsafe for use, every person that has had an amalgam filling placed by a dentist in the US could join a class action law suit against dentists that have ever placed mercury fillings. The way our government and judicial systems are set up, there is no way the governing agencies will change their stance on this.

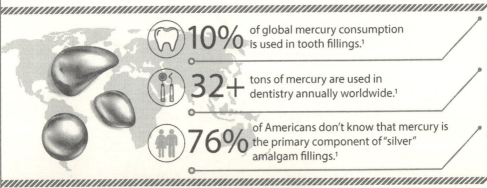

Facts about Mercury

Mercury exposure from dental amalgam is risky for many segments of the population, especially children!

- **10%** of global mercury consumption is used in tooth fillings.[1]
- **32+** tons of mercury are used in dentistry annually worldwide.[1]
- **76%** of Americans don't know that mercury is the primary component of "silver" amalgam fillings.[1]

82.2% of **composites** last at least 10 years.[2]
79.2% of **amalgams** last at least 10 years.[2]

3.7 tons of mercury are discharged each year to Public Owned Treatment Works (POTWs) by dentists, according to EPA studies.[3]

Mercury Pollution: Compared with other sources of mercury pollution, the number of tons consumed globally are:

Lighting	Electrical & Electronic Devices	Measuring & Control Devices	Dental Fillings
120-150 Tons	120-210 Tons	300-350 Tons	313-411 Tons

[1] http://www.toxicteeth.org/CMS Templates/ToxicTeeth/pdf/The-Real-Cost-of-Dental-Mercury-final.aspx
[2] https://www.ncbi.nlm.nih.gov/pubmed/16417916
[3] https://www.epa.gov/mercury/mercury-dental-amalgam

Controversy

The safety of mercury fillings continues to be a very controversial subject. Dentists have lost their dental licenses for speaking out about their beliefs that mercury fillings are toxic. In fact, there are things I can and can't legally say to you about mercury in fillings. Thankfully, there are some undisputed facts:

- Mercury is the most neuro-toxic, non-radioactive element on the planet. It is more neurotoxic than arsenic or lead.[43]

- Dental researchers now concede that mercury vapor is released from unstimulated amalgam fillings 24-hours a day.[44]

- Chewing, brushing, temperature increases and clenching/grinding have been shown to release mercury vapor.[45]

- The FDA and the American Dental Association promote amalgam fillings as standard of care dentistry. Dentists who place amalgam fillings do so in good faith, believing in the efficacy, safety, cost-effectiveness, and longevity of amalgams.[46]

- Norway banned dental amalgam in 2008,[47] Sweden banned it in 2009,[48] and Denmark, Estonia, Finland, and Italy use it for less than 5% of tooth restorations.[49] Japan and Switzerland have restricted or almost banned dental amalgam.[50] France has recommended that alternative mercury-free dental materials be used for pregnant women, and Austria, Canada, Finland, and Germany have purposely reduced the use of dental amalgam fillings for pregnant women, children, and/or in patients with kidney problems.[51]

- A 2005 World Health Organization report warned of mercury: "It may cause harmful effects to the nervous, digestive, respiratory, immune systems and to the kidneys, besides causing lung damage. Adverse health effects from mercury exposure can be: tremors, impaired vision and hearing, paralysis, insomnia, emotional instability, developmental deficits during fetal development, and attention deficit and developmental delays during childhood. Recent studies suggest that mercury may have no threshold below which some adverse effects do not occur." [52]

Metal fillings

So... do mercury fillings affect your health? In that same position paper by the IAOMT in 2016, they presented scores of research pointing to the health implications of mercury fillings. I think this information bears repeating here:[53]

> "*Scientific research demonstrates that dental mercury amalgam exposes dental professionals, dental staff, dental patients, and fetuses to releases of mercury vapor, mercury-containing particulate, and/or other forms of mercury contamination. Dental mercury amalgam is therefore not a suitable material for dental restorations.*
>
> *"Furthermore, mercury vapor is known to be released from dental mercury amalgam fillings at higher rates during brushing, cleaning, clenching of teeth, chewing, etc., and mercury is also known to be released during the placement, replacement, and removal of dental mercury amalgam fillings.*
>
> - *A series of studies demonstrate that urinary mercury concentrations consistently increase as the number of amalgam fillings increases.*
>
> *Numerous studies have also demonstrated that the mercury exposure or concentration increases in the following tissues and situations*
>
> - *Due to chewing, brushing, and/or bruxism*
> - *In exhaled or intra-oral air of persons with amalgam fillings*
> - *In saliva of persons with amalgam fillings*
> - *In blood of persons with amalgam fillings*
> - *In various organs and tissues including the kidney, liver, pituitary gland, thyroid, and brain*
> - *In feces of amalgam bearers*
> - *In amniotic fluid, cord blood, placenta, and various fetal tissues including liver, kidney and brain, in association with maternal amalgam load*
> - *In colostrum and breast milk in association with maternal amalgam load*
>
> *Mercury's damaging influence on the developing brain and neurological system makes dental mercury amalgam fillings an inappropriate material for use in children, pregnant women, and women of childbearing age. In fact, research has repeatedly shown the potential for significant impacts to pregnant women, fetuses, and children as a result of dental mercury."*
>
> *–Position paper by the IAOMT*

The *World Health Organization* (WHO) and Canada's federal department of health (*Health Canada*) have stated that "mercury vapor from dental amalgam is the greatest source of human exposure to mercury in non-industrial settings."[54-55]

The IAOMT also has a stance on how these fillings should be considered in the overall picture of health concerns and problems.

"Additionally, physicians and dentists should, where patients are suffering from pathological states and/or disease of unclear causation, consider in their differential diagnosis whether exposure to mercury released from dental mercury amalgam fillings might be a contributing or exacerbating factor in such adverse health conditions. This is because dental mercury amalgam has been associated with a wide-range of adverse health conditions. It should also be remembered that reactions to mercury exposures vary from person to person, including exposures to dental mercury."[53]

The information above should help you make your decision about your mercury fillings. This choice needs to be yours, and can't be dictated by your dentist or doctor.

When existing amalgam fillings are still in the teeth, chewing and functioning without defects in the fillings themselves, it is your personal choice to have them replaced with other materials, either for health reasons or if you want your teeth to look better. The key is that during the removal, it must be done safely! Continue reading for crucial information about how to have those mercury/amalgam fillings removed.

Mercury fillings are bad for teeth and your body

I've been a mercury-free dentist for nearly 20 years. I made that decision long before I had my own health challenges with mercury. I have never liked what mercury fillings do to your teeth. We are going to go back to basic science here. If you have a bottle with a metal lid that won't open, what do you do? Put the lid under hot water to loosen it. Why do you do that? Because the metal expands when it is heated, and the lid is easier to get off. The same things happens in reverse. When the metal gets cold it shrinks.

Now imagine a mercury filling in a tooth. The filling was intentionally formed like an upside down wedge in the tooth, wider at the bottom and narrower at the top. That was done to help the filling stay in your tooth, because there is no "glue" under a mercury filling.

Continue imagining that upside down wedge as you eat dinner tonight. You start the meal with a delicious soup. It's so hot that you have to blow on each bite. Your metal fillings are expanding with every bite—pushing outward on the walls of the tooth it's wedged into. For dessert, you have apple pie with ice cream on top. That ice cream hits the metal filling and it starts to shrink, pulling away from the tooth.

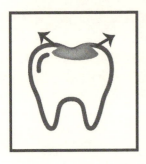 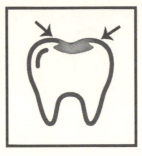

Repeat. And repeat. And repeat every time you eat a meal with hot or cold foods. Eventually the crystals in the tooth walls will start to crack. A gap will also start forming around the edges of the filling as the filling expands and shrinks. Bacteria aren't very big, so they can easily slip into that gap between the tooth and the filling. Can you brush underneath a filling? I don't think so! This leads to new cavities underneath your old mercury filling.

Life span of mercury fillings

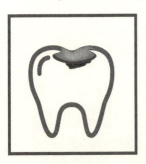

How often does this shrinking and gap formation happen? I have removed thousands of mercury fillings in my career, and I can, from experience, say that 90% of those old fillings have a new cavity underneath. And 100% of the teeth have cracks caused by the filling expanding. There are very frequently structural and physical problems with these old mercury fillings, and that alone is enough to recommend they be replaced. Quite simply, mercury fillings aren't a permanent fix for a tooth. They have an average life-span of 8-12 years before they crack the tooth and leak bacteria around the gap that forms from expansion and shrinking. How long have you had your old fillings?

Like I said, I have been a "mercury-free" dentist for many years, and I still am, but after my health scare, I am now also a "mercury-safe" dentist. There is a difference. The greatest exposure to mercury comes when the old filling is drilled out. Since most mercury fillings will need to be replaced for functional or health reasons, it is essential you have them removed safely. Safe procedures can reduce exposure by up to 90%.

As my practice has grown, I've needed to expand my office. I worked to acquire the lease of the dentist in the neighboring building, and was assessing what I needed to change before I moved in. He had carpet in all of his dental treatment rooms, and the carpet was 15 years old. I realized it was most likely full of mercury and I couldn't work there until that carpet was replaced with laminate or tile that didn't retain mercury.

I was arranging a time for the flooring installers to come and measure to give me a bid, and was explaining to the current dentist why I was replacing the flooring. He said it was fine because he hadn't placed any mercury filling in over 14 years. I told him I wasn't worried about the mercury from fillings being placed. I explained that the mercury in the carpet would come from all of the mercury fillings he had been drilling out for the last 15 years. He was surprised and said, "It's still a problem at that point? You can get mercury in your body from that?"

This dentist has been practicing for over 25 years and is still completely oblivious to the dangers of mercury, and doesn't understand when the mercury exposure occurs. He is part of the great majority of dentists. If you don't visit an intentionally "mercury-safe" dentist, you can be nearly guaranteed that dentist will not remove the fillings safely. It's not negligence or malpractice, it is misinformation and lack of education in the profession of dentistry in general.

SAFE REMOVAL PROCEDURES

What are those procedures? The IAOMT has established the **SMART** (*Safe Mercury Amalgam Removal Technique*)[56] as a standard in the industry. You want a dentist trained in these procedures, and this training is not available in traditional dental school. The dentist must also have special equipment as detailed below:

1. **KEEPING IT COOL** – to reduce mercury release, a lot of water is used to keep the filling cool.

2. **ROCKS, NOT PEBBLES** – the filling is cut into large chunks, which reduces the amount of drilling.

3. **GET IT ALL OUT** – the vacuum must be very strong and placed as close to the tooth as possible. A special device called a *Clean Up* is added to the end of the vacuum tip to help hold the particles in place.

4. **TO BREATHE OR NOT TO BREATHE** – avoid breathing through your mouth during the procedure. It is beneficial to have an alternate source of oxygen on your nose, and an impermeable barrier such as a gold coated mask over the nose.

5. **DAM IT** – a rubber dam won't keep vapors out, but it will keep particles out of your mouth. Must be a non-latex, nitrile rubber dam.

6. **CLEAN UP, CLEAN UP** – everything in the area and around the area should be rinsed very well after removal, and the mouth rinsed with a slurry of chlorella or charcoal.

7. **BIG VACUUM** – a very large vacuum is placed right below the chin to minimize mercury exposure – both in particulate and vapor form.

8. **COVER IT UP** – The dental patient, dentist, dental assistant and any one else in the room should have covers for their body, their head and their face.

What you need to know before and after removal

Removing mercury fillings, even in a safe way, will always produce a temporary increase in a person's exposure to mercury. You need to understand what that mercury will do in your body and what to do to help your body remove it.

Mercury never exists alone in the body. It attaches to other molecules, particularly ones containing sulfur, like the enzymes glutathione and cysteine. You should increase your levels of glutathione before and after removal by supplementing with liposomal glutathione.

There are a few excellent things you can do with your diet in preparation for mercury removal as well.[57]

- Increase sulfur based foods including vegetables from the cruciferous family (cabbage, garlic, broccoli, cauliflower, kale, collards, radishes, wasabi, etc.), which are rich in sulfur. Fermenting these vegetables is the most nutritious way to consume them.
- Garlic is especially powerful, but it's the oil of the garlic that supports detoxification, not the allicin, which is the compound commonly used as an antimicrobial. The take away is that you want the smelly kind of garlic to get the oils, and deodorized garlic is useless for detox! Either eat the garlic raw by chewing it up or purchase a garlic oil supplement.
- Another good binder for heavy metals is chlorella. This is a binder that grabs the mercury and helps remove it from the body. Other binders you'll hear about are clay/zeolites, and pectin. For the kind of mercury found in dental fillings, these bind very weakly, and you would have to take enormous quantities for many years to have much effect, so I don't recommend them.

There are other detox products you can use, but everything should be regulated by your alternative care health provider. Your body cannot handle an increase of these detox substances over a long term, so the treatment should be pulsed – five days on, two days off (to start), working up to ten days on, four days off. If you begin to feel worse, you may be detoxing too quickly.

The body should have the excretory pathways prepared for an increase in mercury after removal as well. The pathways utilized are the kidneys, liver and colon, particularly kidneys for mercury from fillings.

There are many resources online where you can learn more about mercury fillings. Talk to your holistic health care practitioner about whether removal is something they recommend for you.

Chapter Seven:
Fix the Mouth to Heal the Body

I've been to a lot of courses on natural health, and about half way through I start to get uncomfortable. I tire of hearing how everything in the world is bad! Before a couple of hours have passed I have been taught I shouldn't drink milk, eat meat or any GMO or non-organic vegetables. I've been taught it's a bad idea to eat carbs and proteins together, melons with anythings else, or food after 7 pm. That's not all! I've also been told that all the municipal water is contaminated, all the commercial food is devoid of everything good for me, and the health care system as we know it has "gone to pot".

Don't misunderstand what I'm saying; I don't necessarily disagree with any of these health warnings, but I get tired of all the doom and gloom. We have to live in this world, and I choose to be proactive and creative in my approach to the world I've been given. That is what this chapter is about! Enough of all of the controversies and terrible things in dentistry. Let's talk about how to live in the world and have teeth too!

Biomimetic Dentistry

I've shared information about a lot of problems in dentistry, so it is time to talk about what you should seek for in your dental care. If mercury fillings and root canals are bad, what should you do instead? How do you replace them? The answer is simpler than you might think. I'm going to teach you a tool to use when considering dental options. It's called *Biomimetic Dentistry*.

If you look closely at that word, you'll see the root of the word is "mimic". This kind of dentistry mimics a natural tooth and replaces it with something as close to nature as possible. The goal is to return the tooth to its original strength, function and esthetics.

One caution is that the Biomimetic Dental organizations are not entirely holistic in nature. They are focused on replacing dental structures, not necessarily on whole-body health. Biomimetic dentistry, performed along with Holistic and Biologic Dental practices, is the best of all worlds.

Traditional Dental Restorations

Traditional ways to restore teeth focus on the strength of the filling or the crown. The stronger the better, to prevent the dental material from breaking. Unfortunately, this leaves out what is best for the tooth and creates a cycle that isn't too pretty.

There is a sad but very real life cycle of a tooth that happens once it has been traditionally restored.

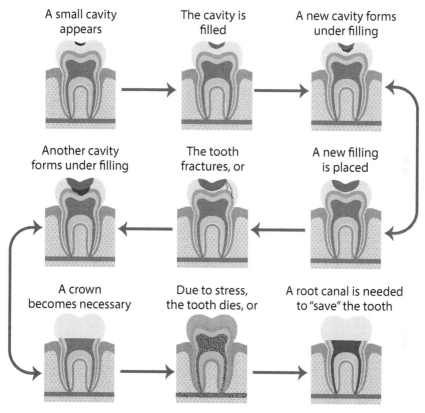

A tooth gets a small cavity and is restored with a strong filling. If it's a mercury filling, it will eventually get a new cavity underneath, which leads to a larger filling. Even new resin fillings often have to be replaced within 10 years of original placement and the filling gets larger each time.

That larger filling weakens the tooth, and sometimes that weakened tooth fractures. The larger filling is also more difficult to place and may not be completely sealed at the edge. The filling then leaks and gets a cavity underneath again.

Another filling may not be possible at this point because of the extent of the tooth structure that has been lost to cavities and breaking. The tooth will now need a crown or an onlay (a porcelain restoration that covers a portion of the tooth rather than the entire tooth like a crown.)

Preparing the tooth for the crown or onlay is stressful on the tooth, and the tooth may die from the stress. The filling and cavity is also deep now, and close to the nerve which also may lead to the tooth dying. Traditionally, a root canal will now be prescribed to "save" the tooth.

As you have learned in previous chapters, that root canal tooth has a high chance of re-infecting, leading to the tooth being lost and either being replaced with a dental implant, or the person choosing to live without the tooth.

Not only is this a sad life cycle for a tooth, it is very costly. Biomimetic dentistry works to intercept this life cycle early in the process and prevent tooth loss and the cost associated with this dental tragedy.

Your tooth needs something that can strengthen the part of your tooth that needs to be stronger, and support and protect the part that is weak. Biomimetic dentistry does just that! If done correctly, 60-80% of traditional crowns and root canals can be avoided.

You read that right. These techniques use a glass/resin mixture called composite, or porcelain, to seal and bond to the tooth. In addition, a holistic dentist will use ozone when placing these restorations to kill any bacteria that may still be living in the tooth. This protects the tooth from further decay, prevents tooth sensitivity, and eliminates stress in the tooth that might cause it to crack or break.

You may have heard of composite fillings and porcelain crowns or onlays. Don't be fooled into thinking they are all alike. There are different ways to use these materials and hundreds of different brands that have very different properties. Fish sticks and a beautifully cooked piece of fish at a fine restaurant are both fish. But the handling, the quality and the preparation are very different. Make sure you are getting the right kind of restoration, performed the right way.

I've seen many composite restorations function for less time than the mercury fillings they replaced. Don't make that mistake. There are, unfortunately, no dental materials that are the exact replacement for tooth structure, but find a dentist that performs Biomimetic Dentistry and you can feel more confident you are getting a restoration that is similar to your natural tooth.

The materials used in the biomimetic method have been intensely researched and have over 25 years of proven clinical success.[2] These restorations will take a dentist more time to complete, and few dentists (fewer than 1%) have received the necessary training. It is worth your time to find a dentist familiar with biomimetic methods to replace fillings and restore your teeth. It's a great question to ask when you call a "biological dentist" from an online search.

Dental Implants

I've talked a lot about possibly needing or wanting to remove teeth. If you do choose to have your tooth removed, how do you replace it? There are four basic options when a tooth has been removed:

> **1. Do nothing.** Leave the space there and don't replace the tooth.
> - *Pros*—This is the least traumatic and least expensive option.
> - *Cons*—Teeth work in relation to one another.
>
>   A. If you remove a top or bottom tooth, the tooth above or below it will move up or down, trying to find something to chew against. This throws the alignment of the bite off. Ask your dentist if the tooth you are having removed will be one that will affect the other teeth if it isn't replaced.
>
>   B. The bone stays stays where it is holding a tooth. When your tooth is removed, the jaw bone that was holding your tooth in place will slowly resorb away. This is particularly true if you have a top back tooth removed. This will make it more difficult to have an implant placed later, and may affect the teeth next to the space as the bone pulls away from those teeth as well.

> **2. Replace it with something removable.** This is called a partial denture or "flipper" if it's replacing a few teeth, or a denture if replacing all of the teeth.
> - *Pros*—This can be removed for cleaning, and can be easily repaired if it breaks. It is the least expensive way to replace the tooth.
> - *Cons*—It does not look or chew like your natural tooth.
>
>   A. Dentures have about a 50% loss in chewing ability from natural teeth.[3] It is difficult to chew things like salad and carrots with dentures.
>
>   B. Many people also don't want to worry about a denture breaking or getting lost at a bad time.
>
>   C. This does not give the bone a tooth to hold, so you will lose jawbone over time. There is an average five-year life span for a denture, because as the jawbone resorbs away the denture gets loose and has to be remade to fit the new shape of the bone.

3. Replace it with something glued in place. This is called a bridge and there are many variations.

- *Pros*—It does not come in and out. It looks and works similar to your natural teeth and can be completed in a few weeks.
- *Cons*—It does negatively affect the teeth holding the bridge.

    A. A bridge puts a lot of pressure on the teeth on both sides of the space that are holding the bridge. This can and often does lead to the supporting teeth being lost as well. In fact, more than 50% of teeth that are holding a bridge are lost within ten years of the bridge being placed. Now you are missing the original tooth and one or both of the teeth next to the missing tooth. You've now turned the one tooth problem into a three tooth problem.[4]

    B. It is more expensive and does not help the bone stay there. It has a ten-year average life span.

4. Replace it with a root-replacing dental implant.

- *Pros*—This is the replacement that looks and works most like your natural tooth. It does not involve or damage any other teeth. It gives the bone a tooth to hold, so the bone does not go away and has a 20+ year life span.
- *Cons*—It takes 6-12 months to complete and is the most expensive option.

    A. There are debates about the long term health implications of dental implants, but most of these debates are in regards to titanium implants (see more information below).

    B. Zirconium implants have been in use for 20 years in Europe, but longer term data is not available.[5]

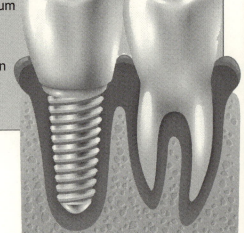

Is a Dental Implant Safe?

I have a dental implant, I replaced my husband's tooth with a dental implant, and that is what I am planning to use to replace my son's missing front teeth when he is done growing and old enough for implants.

There are 30+ year studies showing long term success and safety with dental implants. This success is defined by whether the implant is retained in the mouth and functioning, and there are scores of research articles showing that implants do have a long term retention rate. However, there have not been a lot of definitive studies regarding the health implications of dental implants.

There are some things that cloud this picture even more:

1. Most research has been done testing titanium implants. The first implants were made of titanium, and that has been the standard in dentistry for many years.

2. Recent changes in our environment such as 4G wireless frequencies are impacting the success of the implants. These frequencies cause metals to heat up. Think of a microwave oven. You can't put metals into a microwave because they get too hot when the microwaves hit the metal. The waves in the air from all our wireless devices also hit metals and heat them up by 4-5 degrees Fahrenheit. This small increase heats up the titanium implant and bone surrounding the implant and may lead to bone loss and implant failure. [7]

3. There are many surprising sources of metals in our world today. Metals are hiding in food, personal care supplies like deodorant and shampoo, sun screens, cooking ware, furniture, carpets and more. These metals lead to metal overload in our systems, so the body becomes sensitive to all metals. [8]

After much research and study and training, I am now exclusively placing zirconia implants. These are manufactured from a metal free material called zirconium oxide. It was identified in 1789 by German Chemist Martin Heinrich Klaproth. Zirconium oxide is ivory in color making it similar to the color of the natural tooth. Zirconium can also transmit light, making it very esthetic.

Zirconium oxide implants have outstanding mechanical properties, good stability, a high biocompatibility and a high resistance to scratching and corrosion.[5] Some reasons to choose zirconia implants:

- *Excellent esthetics*
- *Natural white color*
- *Biocompatible*- Research shows no adverse immunologic, tissue or bone reactions to zirconia implants.[9]
- *Preservation of bone*- same success rates as titanium implants.[10]
- *Better gum health*- reduced plaque on implant and tissues, leads to better soft tissue healing and implant success at bone level.[11]
- *Neutral energy*- doesn't interfere with the meridians
- *First choice in patients with titanium allergy.*

Keep reading to find out more about the titanium vs. zirconia debate,[6] but the health and esthetic implications are the reasons I switched over completely.

1. The meridian or shared energy pathways are not blocked by zirconia implants the way they are with titanium.
2. I don't have to be concerned about them heating up when people are using a cell phone.
3. I don't have to cover and mask the gray color of the titanium when I'm restoring them because zirconia implants are white.
4. I don't have to worry about adding to metal overload in a patient's body, which can happen when you add metal to an already toxic body. Environmental metals are found in foods and other products we use every day.
5. I don't have to wonder what that metal is doing to the surrounding bone and tissues and immune system. There are brand new studies that show the immune system never really shuts down around the titanium implants.[12]

While research continues to grow, I am confident in the success of zirconia implants through stories from my patients and thousands of other patients with better health and strong, beautiful zirconia implants. I believe Zirconia dental implants to be the best replacement for teeth today.

Dental Revision

I see an average of four new patients in my practice every day I am working, and these patients come from all over the world. Out of these new patients, half typically are in need of what we call a *"Dental Revision"*.

These people have had a long history of dental work, and have been conscientious about caring for their mouth. Their teeth have followed along the typical path—small filling to larger filling to crown to root canal. They are full of metals and toxins and infection, and they don't know it.

If they don't know it, why are they in my office? Because they have chronic health concerns that no one can find answers for. They have visited practitioner after practitioner, looking for something and someone that can resolve their health concerns and help them get their life back. Often a family member or friend, or one of those health practitioners directs them to our office as a "last hope". We can give them hope because we see lives change every day.

There are some important components that go into a successful dental revision:

1. **Proper nutrition before treatment.** Avoiding processed foods, white sugar and gluten containing grains before a revision is essential. The body must also be fed whole foods that are full of important vitamins and minerals *(see Chapter Five)*.

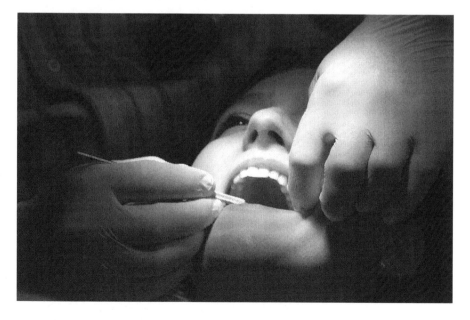

2. **High Vitamin D3 levels.** Vitamin D3 levels must be high for bone to heal after tooth removal and implant placement. The ideal level is over 100 ng/mL from a Vitamin D3 test. (There are now chairside Vitamin D testing units so you can have your levels tested in your holistic dental office. We have one of these units and it saves a patient having to get a blood test)
3. **Proper rest before and after treatment.** In our hurry up world no one wants to slow down, but your body cannot heal without proper rest. The week of the revision should involve a lot of resting, reading, and relaxing and no work.
4. **Therapeutic IV therapy.** High doses of Vitamin C, anti-inflammatory medications, Homeopathic remedies for lymphatic flow and healing and pain relief are all beneficial in a pre- and post-treatment IV.
5. **Same Day Implant Placement.** If possible, implants heal well when placed the same day as the tooth is removed. The body is primed for healing and the bone is preserved.
6. **Biologic Principles in metal and toxin removal and tooth removal and replacement.** All of the principles in this book must be applied to treatment to ensure a successful outcome, dentally and medically.

Chapter Eight:
The Gum and Overall Health Connection

Gums are just like skin, but on the inside. The gums cover and protect the teeth and jaw bone, and keep bacteria and other invaders from getting into the body. They can be damaged and cut, infected, and get diseases just like your skin. If the gums are damaged or diseased, they can't do a very good job of protecting what's below and inside.

These gums are a part of the entire digestive system. The digestive system is a long tube that starts in the sinus cavities and nose and ends at the other end in the rectum. If there is infection anywhere along that system, the entire system affected.

Many people suffer from digestive problems, and a big component of that is your gum health. Gum disease is the most common infection in the world, with estimates up of to 80% of adults having some degree of infection in their gums. If you want to heal your gut and your body, you need to heal your gums.

> Jamie had always been a get-up-and-go kind of woman. Raising three girls of her own, running multiple businesses with her husband, and being a fabulous homemaker were all parts of her normal day.
>
> Over the years she found she wasn't able to do all that she once could, but she thought it was part of getting older. Even though she was careful about what she was eating, she started gaining weight and couldn't get it off. She was slowing down and started having aches and pains. And, the most worrisome part, she lost a few teeth that just got loose and came out.
>
> Not knowing where to go, she visited a traditional dentist, who chastised her for not brushing her teeth well enough. Embarrassed and discouraged, she avoided dentists and doctors for years until she was diagnosed with Type II diabetes and the pain in her body pushed her to do something.
>
> She came to my office and we found Stage Four gum disease along with advanced digestive and arthritic problems that related to the gum disease. After treatment to clean the teeth, kill the microbes with laser and ozone and nutrition that rebuilt her bone and gums, the gum disease resolved. Treatment for her gut also helped her digestive symptoms, symptoms, helped her reverse her diabetes, allowed her to lose some weight and she is back on the road to feeling great again.

Gum Recession

Gum recession is something I check every time I complete an exam for a patient. Why? It's kind of like checking the pressure in your car tires. It's a measuring stick for the health of the mouth, and if you find something a little off, you can quickly correct it before you get a flat tire!

There are two main reasons your gums may start to recede, and neither of them have to do with brushing too hard or getting older. I bet at least 50% of the new patients I see with receding gums tell me a former dentist told them they were brushing their teeth too hard, and that is the reason for the gum problem. The other 50% tell me they are just getting older and receding gums comes with the territory. I'm going to loudly disagree! Let's talk about the real problems which are **Gum Disease** and **An Unbalanced Bite.**

The two basic categories of gum disease are Gingivitis and Periodontitis.

Gingivitis- the official name for the gums is "gingiva". And "itis" always means inflammation. So gingivitis means inflammation of the gums.

- This is the early stage of Gum Disease where the gums bleed easily and are swollen, but the disease has not progressed to the jawbone.

Periodontitis – Remember the ligament that connects your tooth to the bone? It's called the periodontal ligament. This disease is inflammation of the periodontal ligament and the bone beneath. Periodontitis is inflammation of the bone and the gums.

- This is Stage 2-4 gum disease when the disease has progressed into the bone and there has been early to advanced bone loss, threatening the tooth and your overall health.

What causes these diseases?

Bacteria: The bacteria in your mouth like to congregate together. They live in the sticky substance on your teeth and tongue called plaque. The longer they stay in one place, the stickier these colonies get and more bacteria can join them. Just as in any large city, the more bacteria that crowd together, the more garbage they create. It's the garbage (toxins) that inflame the gums.

Pay attention to where the plaque sticks. You'll see it's right around the gumline. If the plaque stays there for longer than a few days, the toxins start to damage the fragile gum tissue. Your body, always on guard, sends it's warriors there to battle this attack. That's what inflammation is, simply your body's reaction to a foreign invader. This inflammation is called gingivitis.

Nutrition: There is another component to gum disease that has very little to do with bacteria. Early in the 19th century, sailors were stricken with scurvy as they sailed across the ocean with a very limited diet. One of the most prominent symptoms of scurvy is bleeding gums and loose teeth. What was missing in these sailor's diets? Vitamin C.[1] If a Vitamin C deficiency could create a disease condition in the gums and bone, it's obvious that nutrition plays a part in gum and bone health.

Other Causes

While bacteria and nutrition are the primary cause of gum disease, there are other factors that contribute. These include:

- **Hormonal changes**, such as those occurring during pregnancy, puberty, menopause, and monthly menstruation, make the blood supply in the gum tissues more inflamed and the gums are more prone to bleeding and soreness.
- **Illnesses** may affect the condition of your gums. This includes diseases such as cancer or autoimmune disease that interfere with the immune system. Diabetes affects the body's ability to use blood sugar, so patients with this disease are at higher risk of developing infections, including periodontal disease and cavities.
- **Medications** can affect oral health, because some decrease the flow of saliva, which has a protective effect on teeth and gums. Some drugs, such as the medication for epilepsy called Dilantin and some heart medications can lead to overgrowth of gum tissue.
- **Bad habits** such as smoking make it harder for gum tissue to repair itself.
- **Family history** of dental disease can be a contributing factor for the development of gingivitis.

Incidence and Progression of Gum Disease

The startling fact is that more than 50% of the adult population in the US has some level of periodontal disease. That means that one out of every two people have this infection. If left untreated, it can lead to inflammation and disease throughout the body.[3]

Although most adults have some level of gum disease, very few people know it's there.[4] Gingivitis is usually not painful. The gums turn red, they bleed when you brush, but they often don't hurt. The early warning system of pain is missing for this disease, which makes it more dangerous.

If the plaque stays there long enough, excess calcium in the blood starts to combine with the plaque and a hard substance called calculus or tartar is formed on the teeth. Now the bacteria are really happy! The calculus is like condos for those bacteria to live in. You can't brush tartar off, so they can live there a long time, continuing to drop their garbage onto the gums.

After a while, the immune system figures out that this invader isn't going away, so it tells the gums to retreat. The periodontal ligament starts to come loose from the tooth, and the gums start to recede down the tooth. This opens up a pathway for the bacterial toxins to get to the bone beneath, which causes the bone to get infected and to start to recede as well. The gums are lost, the bone is lost, and eventually the tooth gets loose and can come out.

What a sorry tale! And most of it happens with no pain. I've often called periodontal disease the silent and deadly killer of teeth. Some warning signs are bleeding gums when you brush, a bad taste in your mouth, loose teeth and bad breath. If you have any of these, run, don't walk to the dentist! You don't have any time to lose!

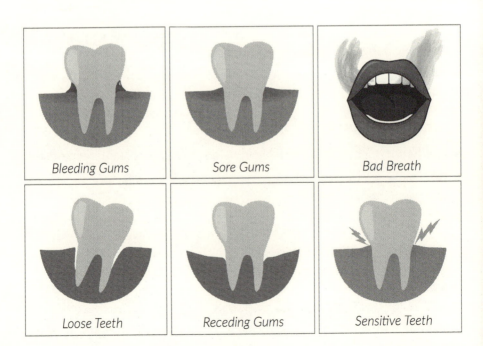

Overall Health Effects of Periodontal Disease

Periodontal Disease is not something to wait on, because decades of scientific research have connected periodontal (gum) disease with other disease-including diabetes, high blood pressure, heart attacks, stroke, kidney and lung disease, cancer, infertility, erectile dysfunction, preterm birth and other pregnancy complications. [5-14]

Some facts:

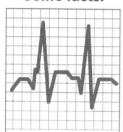

People with periodontal disease have 2x higher risk of dying from heart disease and 3x higher risk of dying from a stroke.

—Mayo Clinic

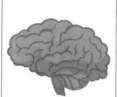

There is a significant connection between periodontal disease and Alzheimer's disease

—Swiss research

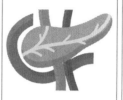

There is a 64% increased risk of pancreatic cancer in those with peri-odontal disease

—Harvard and Dana Farber Cancer Institute

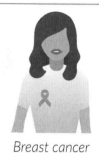

Breast cancer is linked to periodontal disease

—American Cancer Association

Diagnosis of Periodontal Disease

Gum Exam

The health of your gums and bone should be measured at every cleaning, or what we call your "wellness visit". There is a natural pocket between the tooth and gum that is 2-3 millimeters deep. A special measuring tool is placed in this pocket to measure the depth of it. If it is deeper than 3 millimeters, that is a sign that disease has ALREADY happened.

Bone has already been destroyed and the disease has progressed and has caused or is causing damage NOW. You should not wait to begin treatment as each day leads to further effects in the mouth and in the body.

Periodontal Bacteria and Systemic Disease

Cardiovascular Disease

Alzheimer's Disease

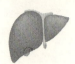
Liver Disease

Fetal Death

Spleen Problems

Infertility & Erectile Dysfunction

Colon Cancer

Osteoporosis

Kidney Disease

Joint Problems

Cancers

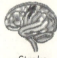
Stroke

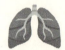
Pulmonary Disease

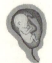
Pre-Eclampsia

Prostatitis

Rheumatoid Arthritis

Coronary Artery Disease

Pre-term Birth

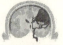
Brain Abscess

Diabetes

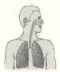
Upper Respiratory Infection

Over 43* areas of health are directly impacted by periodontal disease.

*Bartold 2012

Other diagnostic testing

Bacterial testing: A Phase Contrast Microscope can be used to test for Microbes in your gums. It is not possible to identify specific microbes through this screening, but general types of microbes can be seen, and this can determine numbers of bacteria and the severity of your infection.

DNA testing: There are a few specialized laboratories in the country that can perform DNA test on a bacterial sample taken from the pocket around your teeth. This test can help identify specific microbes so treatment can be targeted specifically.

Blood Testing: Your biologic dentist may recommended Blood testing to identify any nutritional or overall health markers that could be contributing to or influencing your gum and overall health.

Some testing they may request:

- *HbA1c and Fasting Blood Glucose–* this test shows how your body handles sugars
- *Vit D3 (1,25 D hydroxy)–* this test identifies your Vitamin D levels which are essential for healthy bone.
- *Complete Lipid Panel–* commonly known as your cholesterol test, this identifies problems in fatty bone formation.

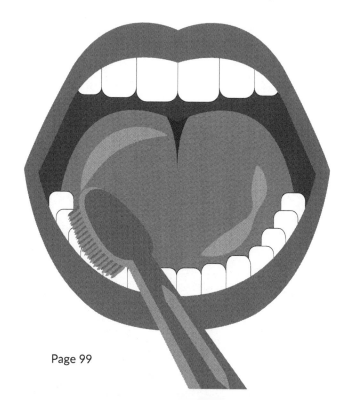

How Periodontal Disease Progresses

Gingivitis: Stage 1

Plaque and bacteria get into the pocket around your teeth and start infecting your gums.

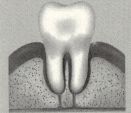

At this stage, there are few signs or symptoms. Some indications of gingivitis include:

- Occasional bad breath
- Redness and swelling of the gums
- Bleeding when flossing
- Gum measurement depths of 2-4 mm

Note: Bone loss has not yet started. The infection is completely reversible.

Slight and Moderate Periodontal Disease: Stage 2, 3

The infection now extends deeper under your gums and is destroying the supporting bone. Your bacteria types change and cause more bone loss as your pockets get deeper.

At this stage, periodontal disease can remain "silent" with few signs and symptoms. Some signs to look for are:

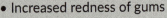

- Increased redness of gums
- Worsening bad breath
- Bleeding on brushing and flossing
- Slight: Gum measurement depths of 4-5 mm
- Moderate: Gum Measurement depths of 6-7 mm
- Pain is unlikely despite the deeper infection and bone loss

Note: At this point, harmful oral bacteria are regularly entering your blood stream and stressing your immune system.

Advanced Periodontal Disease: Stage 4

The infection gets deeper into the gums and bone and the bacteria becomes more dangerous. Your teeth will sustain extensive bone loss and will become loose. Periodontal disease at this stage is no longer "silent". Some signs include:

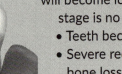

- Teeth becoming loose and coming out
- Severe recession of gums with extensive bone loss
- Raised areas of infection in the gums called periodontal abscesses

- Redness, swelling, and oozing gums
- Cold sensitivity and tooth mobility worsens
- Gum measurement depths of 7+ mm
- Pain when chewing
- Severe bad breath

The infection is now so deep that periodontal surgery or periodontal laser therapy is needed to clean out these deeper pockets of bacteria.

Other Problems that Lead to These Symptoms

There are some things that can mimic gum disease. If the bleeding gums and/or loss of bone is only in certain localized areas, it is very possibly a tooth problem. Have your holistic dentist check:

- Defective dental restorations
- High electric current (galvanism) from metal restorations
- Bite problems
- Mercury fillings in the area.

If the gum disease is more generalized but your teeth are "clean" we will check for health problems, including:

- Depressed immune system
- Low Vitamin C
- Poor diet
- Prescription drug problems
- Hormone imbalances
- pH problems in the gut

Treating Gum Disease

Mechanical cleaning– the bacteria in your mouth creates a sticky layer on your teeth that, if not removed, calcifies and forms tartar that can't be removed on your own. This tartar harbors other, more dangerous bacteria, and has to be removed if your gums and bone are to return to health.

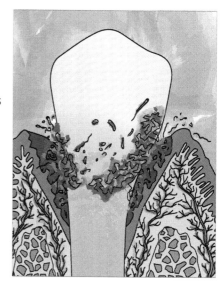

The official name for this treatment is Scaling and Root Planing, and is what is traditionally prescribed if you are diagnosed with gum disease. This cleaning can be done with traditional hand instruments, or with specialized ultrasonic instruments. Both can be utilized to remove all of the hard deposits on your teeth so your gums can heal.

Laser Cleaning and Disinfection- Laser light energy is used to kill microbes over a large area of the infected root, gum tissue and bone. This laser light is tuned into the harmful bacteria in the infected tissue, and up to 99.9% of the disease producing bacteria are killed. In addition to killing the bacteria and infection, the laser also stimulates stem cells in the tissues to form new connective tissues, collagen and bone. Your body can then heal and rebuild these lost tissues.

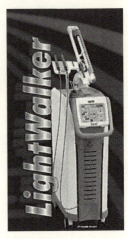

At the end of treatment, a second laser is used to seal the tissues against the tooth root. This protects the pocket from germs and plaque getting back into the area while it is healing.

Ozone Cleaning and Disinfecting- Ozone is one of the most powerful natural oxidizing agents. It kills bacteria, disinfects, stops bleeding and stimulates wound healing. Used in a gas or liquid form, it has been shown to reduce bone loss and infection in 80% of periodontal disease areas, often significantly.

In nature, ozone (O3) occurs from atmospheric oxygen (O2). It develops as a result of ultraviolet light (sun) or electric spark discharge (thunderstorm, lightning) from air oxygen. In medicine, a special device generates a mini thunderstorm in a glass tube, and ozone occurs at the end of the tube. Being a gas, ozone is able to infiltrate the tissues, the smallest fissures, wounds and gum pockets, painlessly and without side effects.

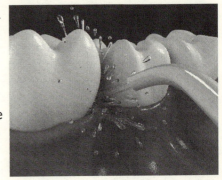

Gum Irrigation- Once the pockets around the teeth are clean, they can be treated with liquid medications to help the tissues heal and regenerate. This procedure is called pocket irrigation and a variety of herbal and other health-stimulating irrigants can be used. I do not recommend using harsh antimicrobials such as Chlorhexidine, because of possible tissue damage.

Frequency of treatment:

After treatment for gum disease and during your healing period, the gum pocket around your teeth is open and deep, inviting bacteria back in. It takes 90 days for that bacteria to repopulate the gum pocket. You should return for gum maintenance to have those pockets irrigated and cleaned again 60-90 days after your treatment, and every 90 days until your condition stabilizes. At these visits, you will have gum exams where all of the pockets are measured. When the pocket depths decrease and the gums are not bleeding, the disease is no longer progressing and you are regenerating gum and bone

Nutrition and Supplementation for Gum Disease Treatment

Vitamins and minerals, particularly the fat-soluble vitamins A, D3, E, K2, are essential to gum and bone health. When a diet is devoid of minerals and high in sugar and processed foods, it causes the body chemistry to be out of balance. Particularly the balance of calcium and phosphorus. This leads to excess calcium in the blood and too little calcium available for the body to use.

In this situation, the body has to borrow. If there is not enough calcium for the essential organs to function, they will borrow it from the bone around the teeth. This sets up a weakened system that will quickly become infected. We see that infection and conclude that gum disease is always an infection caused by bacteria, but poor nutrition set the stage for that infection to occur.

I've seen this delicate balance tip so many times in practice. A patient will have a perfect exam one visit, and six months later, will have gum disease. When we start to ask what's happened in their life in the last six months, we always hear about dietary changes, stress, perhaps illness, and always something that taxed their immune system.

The good news is, I've also seen this in reverse. After addressing the causes of the disease, I've seen bone regrow and gum tissue heal. The body is a masterpiece and has the ability to heal if we provide the tools and materials it needs.

Vitamins	Clinical Features of Deficiency
A	Reduced saliva, gum overgrowth, oral precancerous areas
B1 (Thiamine)	Reduced taste sensation
B2 (Riboflavin)	Sores in the corners of the mouth, oral ulcers, swelling and redness of lips, with vertical cracking, burning mouth
B3 (Niacin)	Burning mouth, swollen red tongue, flattened gums, excess saliva, sores in the corners of the mouth
B6, B12	Dry and sore gums, burning mouth, red beefy tongue, flattened gums, bone loss, bad breath
B9 (Folic acid)	Bad breath, gum inflammation
C	Oral ulcers, sores in the corners of the mouth, gum loss, burning mouth, gingival inflammation, scurvy, delayed gum healing
D	Jaw bone loss, delayed healing after extraction, low jaw bone density
K	Low jaw bone density, delayed healing after extraction, soft tissue bleeding
Minerals	**Clinical Features of Deficiency**
Iron	Red painful tongue, sores in the corners of the mouth, difficulty swallowing
Zinc	Oral ulcers, altered taste sensation, delayed wound healing
Calcium	Low jaw bone density, delayed healing after extraction

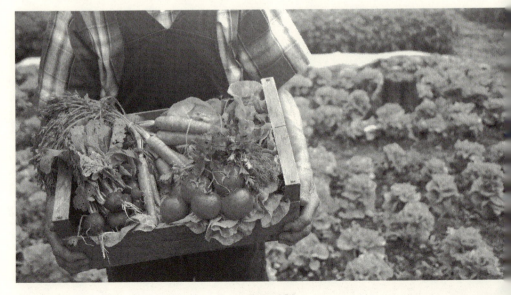

At Home Care after Periodontal Treatment
- Electric Toothbrush twice a day for two minutes
- Water Pik once a day for 2 minutes
- Use Herbal Mouthrinse for one minute (Tooth and Gum Tonic is recommended)
- Tongue Scraper every morning and night

Supplement Recommendations
- Vit D3/K2
- Omega 3 Fatty Acids
- Cell Salts - Calc Fluor, Calc Phos, Silicea
- Dr. Christopher's Complete Tissue and Bone
- Fulvic and Humic Minerals
- Zinc

Gum Disease Prevention

How do you prevent it? Do everything we talked about in the *"Clean The Outside"* section of Chapter Four. If you take those few minutes each day, you can prevent most gum disease. Add to that a healthy dose of Vitamin C and the other fat-soluble vitamins from the foods listed in Chapter Five and your gums are nearly disease-proof.

You can also add a therapeutic mouth rinse

> **Dr. Js Clean and Heal Rinse**
>
> *Ingredients:*
> 1 T baking soda
> 1 t sea salt or Himalayan salt
> 2 C water
> 2 T colloidal or nano silver solution (get online. Favorite source is ASAP 10 PPM Silver Sol Immune System Support from American Biotech Labs.)
>
> *Mix all ingredients in a glass jar. Use 1 oz to swish with after cleaning your teeth.*

Gums and How they Relate to the Bite and the Jaw Joint

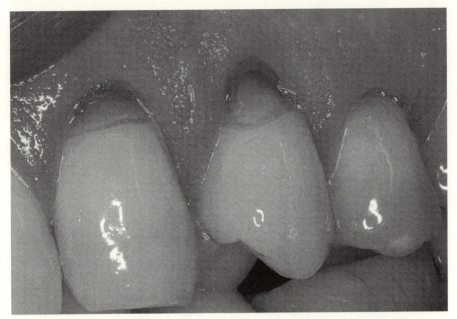

This is the second reason you may get receding gums, and the most misunderstood. If you have gum recession in an area that doesn't have infection, look at the tooth that hits against it when you bite. Does it have recession too? If so, these teeth are hitting too hard and causing the recession. How does this happen? We need to go back to the farm to explain!

My husband loves to build things with green posts. These are metal posts that are pounded deep into the ground. They can be removed and moved to another area, but not without some work. To remove the post, you have to hold on to the top and rock the post back and forth. Eventually the soil around the post starts to pull away and part of the post that is underground becomes exposed. The more rocking you do, the more soil falls away and the more loose the post becomes. Eventually enough soil falls away to allow you to pull the post out of the ground.

The same thing happens with teeth. If teeth hit together too hard or at an angle when chewing, the teeth rock. The gums start to pull away from the teeth as they are rocked and part of the root that was below the gum becomes exposed. The more the rocking happens, the more the gum pulls away and exposes the root. This is called gum recession. The tooth can become loose from this hitting and rocking, and can even be lost.

Most dentists blame this gum recession on you, and say you have been brushing your teeth too hard. When I really started looking at the recession and which teeth it was occurring on, the brushing explanation just didn't make sense most of the time. Why would you brush just a few teeth too hard? Also, those teeth are often sensitive, so wouldn't you stop brushing those teeth too hard if it hurt?

There is damage that can occur from brushing, but the damage happens after the gums have already receded. Remember, the root is covered with cementum that is much softer than enamel. As you brush your teeth, when your brush hits that receded area and the soft root that is exposed, it's like your car tire falling off a soft shoulder on the road. It can dig into the tooth, brushing the root surface away and leaving a hole or divot, which dentists call an abrasion. You weren't brushing too hard; your tooth was too soft.

Why is the recession happening and how to fix it

If the tooth is hitting too hard or at the wrong angle when biting, it needs to be "balanced". This can be done very simply if only one or a few teeth are involved, by minimally reshaping the teeth to fit together better. Often the reshaping needs to happen on old dental work—crowns that were built a little too tall or fillings that were too deep or shallow. After the problem is corrected, the root surfaces can be covered.

This exposed root surface can be covered in one of two ways. You can have a dentist cover the root with filling material to protect it from the toothbrush. You can also have a gum specialist cover the root with gums.

One of the most exciting advances in dentistry today is what I call *Gum Rejuvenation*. Using stem cells and fibrin from your blood, along with a special suturing technique, the existing gums can be moved up the tooth to recover the root. This is an up and coming procedure that avoids some of the problems with traditional gum grafting, and we are using it with great success.

Bite problem that leads to jaw problems

If you have more than just a few teeth with recession, jaw joint problems or pain, or ongoing tooth wear, your solution needs to be more comprehensive.

You've probably heard of TMJ before, as in, "He has TMJ." This is the common way to talk about it, but inaccurate. The jaw joint is called the TMJ (Temporo-Mandibular Joint). A problem with this joint is actually called *TMD (Temporo-Mandibular Dysfunction)* and that is what I am going to call it in this book. Time for another mini-anatomy lesson.

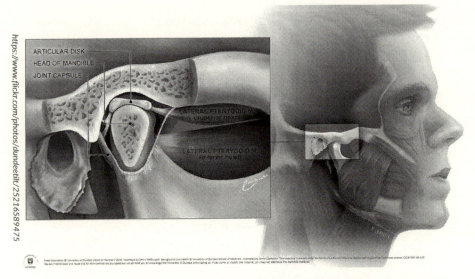

This joint is unique. It is a ball and socket type joint, but it also moves in and out of the joint space. Open and close your mouth and you will see what I mean. When you open, for the first little while the ball just rotates in the socket, then about half way open the ball actually moves forward. There is a slippery piece of cartilage sitting on top of that ball called the disc. It helps the joint slide smoothly when it opens. This is all managed by the muscles in your face and jaw.

There are two kinds of muscles. Opener muscles, which are very small (they only need to pull the joint open) and closer muscles, which are large (they need to be strong to chew through food).

The jaw opening is guided by that disc of cartilage and the sloped bone it slides against. The cartilage can get damaged, moved out of position, or the ligaments that hold it in place can get stretched. When this disc of cartilage is out of place, you hear it pop or click when the jaw opens and closes. Sometimes this is painful and sometimes it is just bothersome.

The jaw closing is guided by the way your teeth fit together, and sometimes the jaw doesn't fit when the teeth do. This can lead to wear and tear problems with the teeth or in the jaw joint. This leads to a dysfunction in the joint and contributes to the majority of TMD issues.[15]

Jaw and teeth imbalances

Imagine you have a rock in your shoe. You try to get the rock out, rattle it around, move your toes to the side, scrunch up your foot... but there is no way to get it out. You move it to a place that bothers you the least and start walking a little differently to avoid the rock. Eventually your knee gets a little sore because you are walking funny, then your hip, and finally your back—all because of a little rock.

This is the most common analogy I use when talking about the jaw not fitting when the teeth fit because it illustrates the problem well.

It is very common to have two "bites". One where the jaw fits–it's all the way in the socket, and one where the teeth fit–they are all the way closed. This difference between the two bites is like that rock in your shoe. Your body doesn't like this discrepancy, so it tries to fix the problem. It clenches the muscles, grinds the teeth together, opens and closes the teeth... but the body can't fix the problem. Eventually, your body figures out how to open and close and chew a little differently to avoid the problem.

Over time, this altered chewing causes your jaw to get a little sore. You wake up with a headache, you get headaches throughout the day, you find it harder to chew hard foods like gum or bagels, your teeth start to wear down, and you get gum recession from the teeth chewing differently. All of this is because your teeth and jaw don't fit together. We call this an "Unbalanced Bite."

These are common signs to watch for:[16]

- Pain in jaw, neck, face, ears or shoulders
- Problems or pain when eating
- Clicking or popping jaw
- Headaches
- Poor sleep
- Dizziness or ringing in ears
- Jaw joint pain
- Muscle spasms or swelling

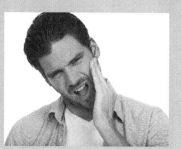

What can you do about it? There is great news! You have options that are short term and long term, and both will bring some measure of relief.

Short-term solution: You can have a special retainer called a *"Deprogrammer"* fabricated that you wear while you sleep. This retainer is not the final fix, but it is the starting point for most TMD treatments and it will stop the damage and will help you feel better almost immediately if you do have a unbalanced bite.

What does the deprogrammer do? It keeps the teeth apart while you wear it, and allows the muscles to relax. It also clears the way so the ball of the jaw joint can go completely back into the socket. This prevents further damage to the teeth or the joint.

How long can I use a deprogrammer? This is not a long term appliance. It can be altered for longer term use after the jaw joint is stable, or you move on to long term solutions.

Long-term solution: There are a few possibilities for long term treatment that are decided by the source of the problem. The first is "Bite Balancing".

Balancing your bite is like balancing your tires–the teeth are strategically reshaped to help them fit together evenly. This is a simple, conservative treatment that fixes the problem about 50% of the time.

If you have extensive tooth wear or broken teeth, bite balancing will not be indicated for you. In the case of worn teeth, the tooth structure needs to be rebuilt with porcelain restorations to reestablish the correct bite. This is called a Dental Rehabilitation. Your dentist can help decide which category you are in.

Braces may also be a solution if your teeth need to be moved for the jaw to seat correctly. There are conservative, non-metal options for braces that are nearly invisible, allowing a lot of adults to get the care they need without the "Brace-face" look of the past. A popular brand is

Invisalign. Make sure to get your orthodontic care through an Orthodontist so he or she can manage any complications that may arise during your treatment.

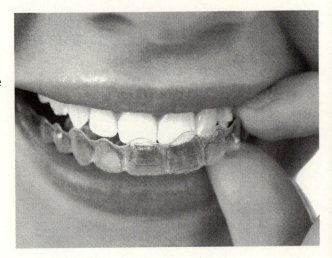

Chapter Nine: Heal What's Possible

This is a step that has been shrouded in secrecy and voodoo. Some books and reports I've read claim that all dentists know how to heal teeth, but that we are keeping it a secret so we can continue to make money off our unsuspecting patients. I'm being facetious, of course. Dentists genuinely want to help people. You don't hear much about healing teeth because most people, dentists included, have not been trained to do it, and don't know how it works. You can heal teeth, and it's not voodoo. It's simple anatomy and chemistry. Most of the rest of the body can heal itself and does so on a regular basis. Of course, the teeth can as well.

Back once again to that anatomy lesson. There are two outside layers in your teeth. The enamel is hard, made up of mineral crystals. The dentin is softer and filled with miles of tubules. Remember what you learned about how cavities form. The first step is minerals being pulled out of the teeth because they are needed elsewhere or dissolved by acids. Once these minerals are gone, the bacteria creep into the enamel.

The second step happens once the bacteria get all the way to the dentin. They infect the dentin, and the infection (decay) spreads quickly because there is a superhighway of tubes filled with fluid to travel along.

You can heal teeth by adding minerals or remineralizing, as long as the decay has not moved into the deeper dentin layer. Once the decay has moved into the

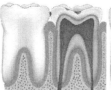
Decay in enamel

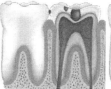
Decay in dentin

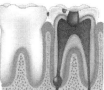
Decay in pulp

dentin, the minerals aren't going to be as effective. This answers the number one question I get about healing teeth, "can any tooth be healed?" Now you know the answer. If the cavity is still in the enamel layer, you can remineralize and heal the tooth. If the cavity has moved into the dentin, most times you will need to have that decayed dentin removed to stop the spread of the cavity, and then fill the hole with resin filling material or cover the area over with porcelain depending on how large the hole the decay created.

How do you know if the cavity has spread to the deeper dentin layer? It can be seen on an xray, and cavity detecting lasers can tell how deep the cavity is. Both require a trip to the dentist, but now you know what to ask.

There are some new technologies to "arrest" or stop decay that have had mixed results. Keep watching as dentistry pursues more preventative measures.

How Can You Remineralize Teeth?[1]

Two basic things need to happen. You need to reduce the acid in your mouth to prevent further mineral loss, and you need to strengthen the tooth. Let's talk about how you can accomplish both of those things.

Acid and saliva

Every time you eat, your mouth becomes more acidic. It's the first step in the digestive process and necessary to help digest your food. In a healthy mouth and body, saliva quickly clears the food and acid out, and helps the mouth return to a neutral level. In fact, saliva is a very important factor in remineralization. It is what carries the minerals back to your teeth.

The saliva returns your mouth to a neutral level if given enough time. This is where frequent snacking or sipping gets you in trouble. If I see a patient with a lot of dental decay, I ask them about their snacking and sipping habits. Some people tell me they drink soda, but only one can a day, sipping it slowly throughout the day. They think they are doing a good thing, but that's the most damaging way to drink a sugary drink (diet soda and fruit juice included.)

I tell them if they are going to drink soda, they should swig the entire can and be done with it. Why? Every time that soda enters the mouth, it makes the mouth more acidic. If someone sips soda every 45 minutes, the saliva never has long enough to help the mouth recover from that acid attack. The enamel will dissolve.

The other problem is too little saliva. Medications will often cause dry mouth as a side effect. I've seen a patient with a healthy mouth one visit return with ten cavities the next. What changed? They were put on a blood pressure medication and had a dry mouth as a result. Without that protective and remineralizing saliva, the teeth dissolved and the bacteria moved in to finish the job.

How to reduce acid in your mouth

The first way to reduce acid in your mouth is to stop putting it there. I'm not talking about a tomato or pineapple with a meal. Your saliva will take care of that. I'm talking about acidic drinks and overuse of acidic foods.

My sons did a science fair project studying the effect of different drinks on tooth enamel. They soaked extracted teeth in seven different liquids and then measured the amount of enamel loss. Their findings were interesting, and I think they will surprise you. If you are wondering about the validity of a high school science fair project, I've found research from dental journals that shows the same thing. This chart lists the most acidic (therefore most destructive) drinks from least acidic to most acidic:[2]

Beverage	Acid pH
Water	7.0 (neutral)
Sports Drinks	
Skinny Water Goji Fruit Punch	3.67 (0.01)
Activ Water Power Strawberry Kiwi	3.38 (0.03)
Sobe Life Water Mango Melon	3.29 (0.01)
Dasani Grape	3.05 (0.01)
Dasani Strawberry	3.03 (0.01)
Propel Berry	3.01 (0.00)
Gatorade Lemon-Lime	2.97 (0.01)
Activ Water Focus Dragonfruit	2.82 (0.04)
Powerade Orange	2.75 (0.02)
Activ Water Vigor Triple Berry	2.67 (0.01)
Fruit Juices and Fruit Drinks	
V8 Fusion Pomegranate Blueberry	3.66 (0.00)
Juicy Juice Apple	3.64 (0.01)
Minute Maid Natural Energy Mango Tropical	3.34 (0.02)
CapriSun Surfer Cooler	3.08 (0.00)
V8 Splash Strawberry Kiwi	2.99 (0.01)
Crystal Light Fruit Punch	2.96 (0.02)
Sunny D Smooth	2.92 (0.01)
Tropicana Twister Orange Strawberry Banana Burst	2.89 (0.01)
Ocean Spray Cran-Pomegranate	2.72 (0.01)
Kool-Aid Mix Cherry	2.71 (0.00)
Barber's Lemonade	2.69 (0.00)
Sobe Black and Blueberry Brew	2.69 (0.00)
Tropicana Juice Beverage Cranberry	2.59 (0.00)
Sodas	
Canada Dry Club Soda	5.24 (0.03)
A&W Root Beer	4.27 (0.02)

A&W Cream Soda	3.86 (0.01)
7UP Diet	3.48 (0.00)
Mountain Dew Code Red	3.27 (0.01)
Sprite	3.24 (0.05)
Dr Pepper Diet	3.20 (0.00)
Coca-Cola Diet	3.10 (0.05)
Sierra Mist	3.09 (0.02)
Mellow Yellow	3.03 (0.00)
Sunkist Orange	2.98 (0.01)
Coca-Cola Zero	2.96 (0.03)
Hawaiian Punch (Fruit Juicy Red)	2.87 (0.01)
Pepsi	2.39 (0.03)
Coca-Cola Caffeine Free	2.34 (0.03)
Energy Drinks	
Fuel Energy Shots Lemon Lime	3.97 (0.01)
Redbull regular	3.43 (0.01)
Nitrous Monster Super Dry	3.46 (0.00)
Killer Buzz Sugar Free	3.36 (0.00)
Redline Xtreme Triple Berry	3.24 (0.01)
Full Throttle Blue Agave	3.10 (0.01)
No Fear Sugar Free	3.06 (0.01)
Jolt Blue Bolt	2.96 (0.00)
Rockstar Recovery	2.84 (0.01)
Redline Peach Mango	2.74 (0.02)
24:7 Energy Cherry Berry	2.61 (0.01)
Tea and Coffee	
Starbucks Medium Roast	5.11 (0.05)
Red Diamond Tea Fresh Brewed Sweet Tea	5.04 (0.02)
Milo's Famous Sweet Tea	4.66 (0.02)
Admiral Iced Tea Sweet Tea	3.76 (0.01)
Snapple Diet Raspberry Tea	3.39 (0.02)
Lipton Green Tea With Citrus Diet	2.92 (0.00)
Nestea Red Tea Pomegranate and Passion Fruit	2.87 (0.01)
Arizona Iced Tea	2.85 (0.03)

Teeth start to dissolve at a pH of 5.5. The acid is more important than the sugar in the destruction of tooth structure. Sorry diet soda drinkers, that artificial sweetener will do nothing to protect the health of your teeth. In my son's study they also tested *Crystal Light* diet drink. It was found to be the most destructive of any of the liquids they tested. It's the acid, not the sugar!

Other sources of acid

Some food may be surprising in their acidity. We know lemon juice is acidic, but most fruit juices are as well (listed least to most acidic).

Beverage	Acid pH
Fruit	
Tomatoes	4.30-4.90
Oranges	3.69-4.34
Peaches	3.30-4.05
Apples	3.30-4.00
Pineapples	3.20-4.00
Blueberries	3.12-3.33
Grapefruits	3.00-3.75
Pomegranates	2.93-3.20
Grapes	2.90-3.82
Blue Plums	2.80-3.40
Limes	2.00-2.80
Lemon Juice	2.00-2.60

Some other surprising foods that are acidic

- Sweeteners, such as sugar, molasses, maple syrup, processed honey and aspartame
- Condiments, such as mayonnaise, soy sauce, and vinegar
- Hard and processed cheeses
- Coffee

The second way to reduce acid is to make sure you give your saliva time to do it's work. Wait at least a couple of hours between eating or drinking anything other than water or simple herbal tea.

How to Replace Minerals in the Teeth

The enamel in your teeth acts like a tiny receiving dock. Your teeth are in constant flux, with the saliva removing and returning minerals throughout the day and night. As long as more minerals are being deposited than removed, your teeth will stay healthy.

Must be able to receive minerals

On that receiving dock, if the doors to the warehouse are closed, it doesn't matter how many minerals are delivered. To keep the "doors" open on your tooth so the minerals can get in, the tooth must be clean.

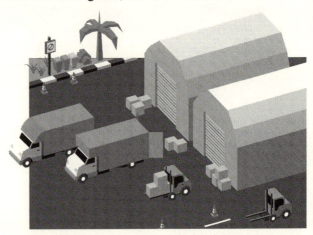

Regular cleaning with the 7 minute regimen in Chapter 4 will do the trick, but make sure you aren't using a tooth care product that contains glycerine. Glycerine will coat the tooth and the minerals can't get in. Most commercial toothpastes contain glycerine, which is one big reason to avoid them.

Minerals must be present in the saliva

When the saliva comes to make a delivery, it needs to be full of minerals to spare. First check that your digestive system is absorbing properly with the *Baking Soda Test* found at the end of Chapter Five. Once you are absorbing properly, you need to add more minerals to your system. Use the following ideas to add more minerals to your system.

I grew up in a backwoods area of Utah, in a little town called Cleveland. It was a great place to live—our back yard bordered onto a field that felt like it went on for days. There were cows to chase around, open ditches to swim in, trees to climb... and asparagus.

I never saw asparagus in the store in those days, but it was growing wild all along the ditch banks behind our house. The fields weren't ours, but I guess we thought the asparagus was! All spring my mom would send us out with a bag to pick whatever we could find.

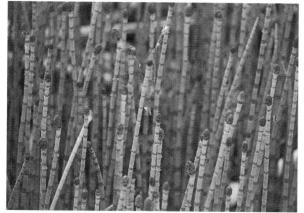

If you've roamed ditch banks before, you're sure to have seen another prolific wild plant that we called Snake Grass. It's the cool grass that looks like a green tube, with sections that you can take apart and put back together. I didn't think it was useful for anything, but boy was I wrong!

Snake Grass, or Horsetail, is chock full of silica. Silica is a crystal that can be incorporated into the teeth and make them stronger. Since only six hundred people live in Cleveland, and you most likely aren't one of them, you are going to have to get your silica another way than along the ditch bank! You can take a supplement of Horsetail. Dosages will be summarized below in the *Tooth Remineralization Game Plan*, below.

Don't take too much calcium

We've all been taught to take calcium supplements to build your bones...and teeth. But that's not the whole story. Let's take a journey with that calcium pill you took this morning. Down the hatch it goes, through the stomach and into the intestines. It is then absorbed through the intestinal wall and enters the bloodstream. Looking good so far. The bones are needing a little extra calcium today, so the calcium heads over there and it's REJECTED! That's right – bones tend to reject calcium – the first problem with a calcium supplement.[3]

The calcium needs to be accompanied by two friends, Vitamin D3 and Vitamin K2, to be effectively absorbed and used. Without these helper nutrients, calcium builds up in the plaque in coronary arteries and creates stones in organs. In fact, without adequate Vitamin D3 levels, your body will only absorb 10-15% of the calcium from your diet or supplements. The Vitamin K2 is then needed to direct that calcium to the proper location. Think of the Vitamin D3 as the gatekeeper and Vitamin K2 as the traffic cop. The gate can be open, but without direction there is chaos. Both are essential for healthy teeth.

Tooth Remineralization Game Plan

1. **Stop taking too much calcium.** 500 mg per day is plenty.
2. **Take a Vitamin D3/K2 supplement.** 5,000-10,000 IU Vit D3 with 300-500 mcg Vit K2 per day. (this is not the same as Vit K1 which affects clotting.)
3. **Make sure the foods you eat actually have nutrients in them.** Refined sugar and flour have none. If you want to build strong teeth and bones, you have to eat the stuff that will build them. Chapter Five explains this in detail.
4. **Take a Silica/Horsetail supplement.** This is easy and inexpensive. For teeth repair and building, 1,500 mg per day. For maintenance, 500 mg per day. It can be found at most health food stores or online.

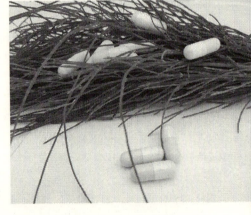

5. **Calc Fluor and Calc Phos.** These are two of the twelve homeopathic cell salts that form the building blocks of the body. They are often lacking in today's diet and are especially important to strengthen teeth and bones in growing children and expecting women. Every member of the family can take them in the dosage listed on the bottle daily. Hylands is a good brand.

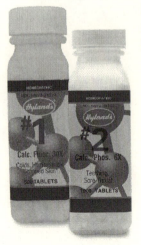

Chapter Ten: Protect Your Body and Health

Every year millions of people will suffer problems from preventable illnesses. You and I are probably in that group. Some simple symptoms we write off as stress or lack of sleep. Other more serious conditions like arthritis, kidney damage, auto-immune diseases and heart disease can spring up for no obvious reasons and have us scratching our heads.

As I said in earlier chapters, physicians have estimated that up to 80% of all illness is related entirely or partially to problems in the mouth. Many health care providers seem to forget that there is a person attached to every tooth!

I had a recent new patient visit that rocked my understanding of this. She had suffered from sinus problems for years, and felt tired and a little sick all the time. She had visited numerous doctors and dentists, and no one had any answers for her. On her first visit, I noticed something suspicious on the routine xray we took. I told her I needed to see her sinus and root area more clearly and recommended a CT scan.

I was shocked with what I found. Three-fourths of her left sinus was filled with a large mass. It was connected to two failing root canals and had caused two additional teeth to die. I don't know how she was breathing and functioning. She has since had the mass removed and we are waiting on the results of the biopsy. She already has more energy than she has had in years and feels like she is getting her life back. Teeth can affect your health in a big way—locally and systemically.

Shared Energy Channels or Meridians

I was introduced to energy channels or meridians years ago, but didn't understand what they were all about. Patients would ask me about them, and I would dance around the subject. At a course by Dr. Jerry Tennant MD, a pioneer in chronic disease prevention and treatment, I finally came to understand the true nature of these energy channels. I learned how they work and how they relate to dentistry, and I want to simplify the concept for you as well.

We are very accustomed to electricity and how it runs the appliances and devices we use every day. What not everyone realizes is that our bodies also run on electricity, including our heart and brain. If you have an EKG to test your heart it is measuring your heart's electrical activity. When you have an EEG it is testing the electrical activity in your brain.

If I want to dry my hair, I plug the hair dryer into an electrical outlet. When my cell phone battery dies, I plug it into an outlet to recharge it. How do we get energy to our body, and how do we recharge when that energy is running low? We don't plug into the wall, but we have to get energy from somewhere.

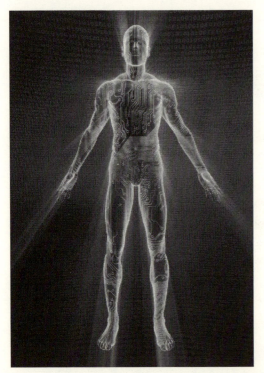

We recharge through our food and our muscles. Food is literal fuel for our bodies, which is why it is so important to eat food that is full of nutrients. Energy is also created when we move our muscles. Each muscle is "wired" to a particular group of organs and functions in our body. This wiring runs along the outside of the muscle called the fascia, connecting organs together in a shared energy channel. Each channel also passes through a tooth or two adjacent teeth.

Three thousand years ago the Chinese discovered this "wiring" and called this energy *Chi* (also spelled "Qi"). They called these shared energy channels that were wired together "meridians" and knew how to access and affect these meridians through acupuncture or acupressure points on the skin.[1]

In the early 1940s, Dr. Reinhold Voll,[2] a medical doctor, anatomy professor and acupuncturist was able to document the meridians the Chinese had known about for centuries. He developed a simple measuring device to measure electric flow on the skin. Using the Chinese acupuncture points, he was able to determine if the energy flow was normal, too strong or too weak along the specific energy channels.

How does this apply to dentistry? As long as this energy flows freely through the shared energy channel or meridian, a body stays healthy. However, once the flow of energy is blocked, the system is disrupted and pain or illness will occur.

Loneliness, Acute Grief, Humiliated, Trapped, Inhibited, Greed, Not Lovable	Anxiety, Self-Punishment, Broken Power, Hate, Low Self-Worth, Obsessed	Chronic Grief, Sadness, Controlling, Feeling Trapped, Dogmatic, Compulsive, Uptight	Anger, Resentment, Frustration, Blaming, Incapable To Take Action, Manipulative	Fear, Shame, Guilt, Broken Will, Shyness, Helpless, Deep Exhaustion	Fear, shame, guilt, broken will, shyness, helpless, deep exhaustion	Anger, resentment, frustration, blaming, incapable to take action, manipulative	Chronic grief, sadness, controlling, feeling trapped, dogmatic, compulsive, uptight	Anxiety, self-punishment, broken power, hate, low self-worth, obsessed	Loneliness, Acute Grief, Humiliated, Trapped, Inhibited, greed, not lovable
Duodenum, Middle Ear, Shoulder, Elbow, CNS S-I Joint, Foot, Toes	Sinus: Maxillary Oropharynx, Larynx	Sinus: Paranasal And Ethmoid, Bronchus, Nose	Sinus: Sphenoid Palatine Tonsil, Hip, Eye, Knee	Sinus: Frontal Pharyngeal Tonsil, Genito-Urinary System	Sinus: Frontal Pharyngeal Tonsil, Genito-Urinary System	Sinus: Sphenoid Palatine Tonsil, Hip, Eye, Knee	Sinus: Paranasal And Ethmoid, Bronchus, Nose	Sinus: Maxillary Oropharynx, Larynx	Duodenum, Middle Ear, Shoulder, Elbow, CNS S-I Joint, Foot, Toes
	Right Breast							Left Breast	
Heart, Small Intestine, Circulation/ Sex, Endocrine	Pancreas Stomach	Lung Large Intestine	Liver Gallbladder	Kidney Gallbladder	Kidney Gallbladder	Liver Gallbladder	Lung Large Intestine	Stomach Spleen	Heart, Small Intestine, Circulation/ Sex, Endocrine
1	2, 3	4, 5	6	7, 8	9, 10	11	12, 13	14, 15	16
32	31, 30	29, 28	27	26, 25	24, 23	22	21, 20	19, 18	17
Heart, Small Intestine, Circulation/ Sex, Endocrine	Lung, Large Intestine	Pancreas, Stomach	Liver, Gallbladder	Kidney Bladder	Kidney Bladder	Liver, Gallbladder	Spleen, Stomach	Lung, Large Intestine	Heart, Small Intestine, Circulation/ Sex, Endocrine
Shoulder, Elbow Ileum, Middle Ear, Peripheral Nerves, S-I Joint, Foot, Toes	Sinus: Paranasal and Ethmoid, Bronchus, Nose	Sinus: Maxillary Larynx, Lymph, Oropharynx, Knee	Sinus: Sphenoid, Palatine Tonsil, Hip, Eye, Knee	Sinus: Frontal, Ear, Pharyngeal Tonsil, Genito-Urinary System	Sinus: Frontal, Ear, Pharyngeal Tonsil, Genito-Urinary System	Sinus: Sphenoid, Palatine Tonsil, Hip, Eye, Knee	Sinus: Maxillary Larynx, Lymph, Oropharynx, Knee	Sinus: Paranasal and Ethmoid, Bronchus, Nose	Shoulder, Elbow Ileum, Middle Ear, Peripheral Nerves, S-I Joint, Foot, Toes
	Right Breast							Left Breast	
Loneliness, Acute Grief, Humiliated, Trapped, Inhibited, Greed, Not Lovable	Chronic Grief, Overcritical, Sadness, Contolling, Feeling Trapped, Dogmatic, Compulsive, Uptight	Anxiety, Self-Punishment, Broken Power, Hate, Low Self-Worth, Obsessed	Anger, Resentment, Frustration, Blaming, Incapable to Take Action, Manipulative	Fear, Shame, Guilt, Broken Will, Shyness, Helpless, Deep Exhaustion	Fear, Shame, Guilt, Broken Will, Shyness, Helpless, Deep Exhaustion	Anger, Resentment, Frustration, Blaming, Incapable to Take Action, Manipulative	Anxiety, Self-Punishment, Broken Power, Hate, Low Self-Worth, Obsessed	Chronic Grief, Overcritical, Sadness, Contolling, Feeling Trapped, Dogmatic, Compulsive, Uptight	Loneliness, Acute Grief, Humiliated, Trapped, Inhibited, Greed, Not Lovable

Acumeridian Tooth-Organ Relationships
(with autonomic/neuropeptide emotion correlations)

Abriged from various sources by Dr. Ralph Wilson www.integrativehomeopathy.com

Imagine a river flooding and backing up, destroying everything in its path, or a power grid short-circuiting that causes blackouts across the area that the power grid supplies power to.

If a tooth is infected or inflamed, or contains metals that interfere with electrical current, the natural flow of energy is blocked along the entire pathway it is on. When this occurs, any organ system connected to the tooth's meridian pathway can be affected in a negative way and eventually lead to poor health and or chronic illness. It either backs up or short circuits.[3]

It can also work in the reverse. If there are systemic problems on the shared energy meridian with a tooth, it may affect the health of the tooth. Holistic or biological dentistry works to eliminate the imbalances and restore the mouth and the body to health. This is why systemic conditions like digestive problems, joint pains, fatigue, headaches, sinus infections, heart disease and even cancer may correct themselves after the dental infection, inflammation and toxins are removed.

How Periodontal Disease Affects the Body

We talked at length in chapter eight about periodontal disease and how it is a silent killer of teeth. It's also a silent killer... period. If you have periodontal disease, that alone is a sign that your body's defenses are weak. That's a big problem, because the harmful bacteria living in the pocket around the tooth don't stay there. The same blood that flows throughout your entire body flows through your gums.

Periodontal bacteria have been found all over the body, including in plaque in the arteries around the heart. An article by Bradley Bale, MD, and Amy Doneen, ARNP published in the *Postgraduate Medical Journal* in April 2017 demonstrates that bacteria from dental infections directly cause heart attacks and strokes. Their article, "High-risk Periodontal Pathogens Contribute to the Pathogenesis of Atherosclerosis," is a landmark publication. Before this study, hundreds of research articles had shown that dental bacteria contributed to heart disease. This new study shows that dental bacteria CAUSE heart disease.[4] From their research, Bale and Doneen concluded that dentists now have the added responsibility of diagnosing and treating dental disease not only to help patients save their teeth and gums, but also to potentially save their lives.

Ulcers— Ulcers have recently been found to be caused by bacteria, not by acid. The culprit is H-pylori bacteria, and the main source is from the mouth. If you have more of these bacteria because of periodontal disease, they can travel from the mouth to the stomach by simply swallowing.

Stroke— Studies have shown that people with periodontal disease have a 200% greater risk of having a stroke.

Birth weight— Alarming studies show that mothers with periodontal disease have a higher risk of low birth weight babies, which leads to many post-birth complications. The bacteria also cross the placental barrier which could lead to infection in the baby.

Senior health— The leading cause of death in a care center is pneumonia. There is a study that shows those with periodontal disease are at a higher risk of developing pneumonia. In fact, periodontal bacteria have been found in the lungs.

Fluoride, Friend or Foe?

All dental students are taught that fluoride prevents cavities. All school children are taught the same thing. I remember the monthly dosing of little green or pink cups of fluoride "swish" in school as I was growing up. This is a proven fact, right? Wrong.

In the Spring of 2016, the *Harvard Public Health* periodical published an insightful article about fluoride, without the hype and intrigue that often goes along with this topic. They reported that, *"Since the mid-1940s, compounds containing the mineral fluoride have been added to community water supplies throughout the U.S. to prevent tooth decay. Health concerns expressed by opponents have largely been dismissed until recently. Now, evidence is mounting that in an era of fluoridated toothpastes and other consumer products that boost dental health, the potential risks from consuming fluoridated water may outweigh the benefits for some individuals. Last summer, for the first time in 53 years, the U.S. Public Health Service lowered its recommended levels of fluoride in drinking water."*[5] It's illegal to dump fluoride into our lakes and rivers, but it's recommended to put it into our drinking water and toothpaste.

Why fluoride?

Research in the early 1900s linked high levels of natural fluoride in the water to less tooth decay. Seeking to replicate this in areas that didn't have natural fluoride, Grand Rapids, Michigan, became the first community 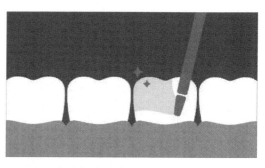 in the world to add fluoride to tap water in 1945. Studies of the effects of this addition showed significantly lower levels of tooth decay in children, so water fluoridation spread, being touted as one of the ten great public health achievements of the 20th century.

However, research flaws have been discovered, and health concerns have surfaced after this widespread water fluoridation. In June 2015, the *Cochrane Collaboration*—a global independent network of researchers and health care professionals known for rigorous scientific reviews of public health policies—published an analysis of 20 key studies on water fluoridation. They concluded that early scientific investigations on water fluoridation (most were conducted before 1975) were deeply flawed.

"We assessed each study for the quality of the methods used and how thoroughly the results were reported. We had concerns about the methods used, or the reporting of the results, in the vast majority (97%) of the studies. For example, many did not take full account of all the factors that could affect children's risk of tooth decay or dental fluorosis. There was also substantial variation between the results of the studies, many of which took place before the introduction of fluoride toothpaste. This makes it difficult to be confident of the size of the effects of water fluoridation on tooth decay or the numbers of people likely to have dental fluorosis at different levels of fluoride in the water." This may explain why countries that do not fluoridate their water have also seen big drops in cavity rates.

How does it work?

Since you've learned about tooth anatomy in Chapter Two, you're going to understand fluoride very well. The mineral is structurally very similar to calcium, so if it is present in the saliva, it will be pulled into the enamel, taking the place of calcium. It forms a harder crystal that is more resistant to bacterial attack. Sounds great, so why have researchers raised flags on fluoride and its safety? There are some large health and dental problems with fluoride, too.

- Teeth and bones with fluoride containing crystals are more brittle.
- Fluoride kills an enzyme needed to uptake calcium into the teeth and other organs.
- Fluoride interferes with hormones, which interferes with tooth remineralization and hormone pathways throughout the body, particularly the Thyroid hormone pathways.
- Too much fluoride causes many cosmetic and systemic problems.

Research against fluoride

Plenty of scientists have spoken out about fluoride and the way it is used in our water supply. Some of the early opponents were Dr. William Marcus, Senior Science Advisor to the EPA Office of Water, and Dr. Phyllis Mullenix, a Harvard researcher. They were both fired after sounding the alarm on fluoride as a neurotoxin, and its causes and effects on rats, including hyperactivity, memory problems and ADD/ADHD. [6, 7]

Sources of fluoride

Although fluoride exists naturally in our world, human exposure to fluoride has markedly increased since the 1940s.

Products that may contain added fluoride include the following:	
Fluoridated municipal water	Beverages made with fluoridated water
Dental cements with fluoride	Dental fillings with fluoride
Dental gels with fluoride	Dental varnishes with fluoride
Floss with fluoride	Fluoride drugs ("supplements")
Food (that contains or has been exposed to fluoride)	Mouthwash with fluoride
Pesticides with fluoride	Pharmaceutical drugs with perfluorinated compounds
Stain resistant and waterproof items with PFCs	Toothpaste with fluoride
Fluoride is also in the air, soil, water and plants from manufacturing and other industries.[8,9,10,11]	

How Fluoride Affects Health

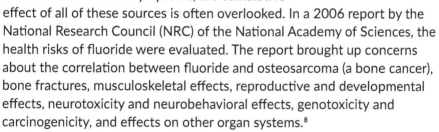

While the impact of fluoride from one of these sources may not be enough to cause health problems and their related symptoms, the cumulative effect of all of these sources is often overlooked. In a 2006 report by the National Research Council (NRC) of the National Academy of Sciences, the health risks of fluoride were evaluated. The report brought up concerns about the correlation between fluoride and osteosarcoma (a bone cancer), bone fractures, musculoskeletal effects, reproductive and developmental effects, neurotoxicity and neurobehavioral effects, genotoxicity and carcinogenicity, and effects on other organ systems.[8]

The following chart from the IAOMT in their 2017 fact sheets includes some of the specific health conditions that have been associated with fluoride exposure:[12]

Adverse Human Health Conditions Associated with Fluoride Exposure	
Acne and other dermatological conditions	Arterial calcification
and arteriosclerosis	Bone weakness and risk of fractures
Cancer of the bone, osteosarcoma	Cardiac failure
Cardiac insufficiency	Cognitive deficits
Dental fluorosis	Diabetes
Early puberty in girls	Electrocardiogram abnormalities
Harm to the fetal brain	Hypertension
Immune system complications	Insomnia
Iodine deficiency	Lower fertility rates
Lower IQ	Myocardial damage
Neurotoxic effects, including ADHD	Osteoarthritis
Skeletal fluorosis	Temporomandibular joint disorder (TMD)
Thyroid dysfunction	

Too Much Fluoride = Dental Fluorosis

Fluoride concentrates in the bone and teeth, and too much fluoride leads to dental fluorosis, a condition in which the teeth are mottled with brown and white areas. This is permanent damage that occurs in the developing enamel. The teeth that are affected are brittle and break easily.[13]

It has been known since the 1940s that overexposure to fluoride causes this unsightly damage, which can range from very mild to severe. Dental fluorosis is also recognized as the first visible sign of fluoride toxicity.

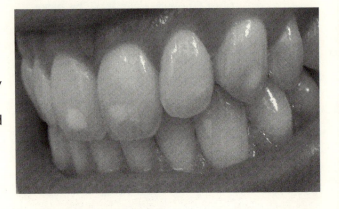

The IAOMT fact sheet also stated that, "According to 2010 data from the Centers for Disease Control and Prevention (CDC), 23% of Americans aged 6-49 and 41% of children aged 12-15 exhibit fluorosis to some degree. These drastic increases of dental fluorosis were a crucial factor in the Public Health Service's decision to lower its water fluoridation level recommendations in 2015."

There are fluoride-free strategies that can prevent dental caries. Given the current levels of exposure, it has become a necessity to reduce and work toward eliminating avoidable sources of fluoride exposure, including water fluoridation, fluoride-containing dental materials, and other fluoridated products.

The Harvard Public Health article concluded that, "We should recognize that fluoride has beneficial effects on dental development and protection against cavities. But do we need to add it to drinking water so it gets into the bloodstream and potentially into the brain?" There is enough research to the contrary to answer this question with a resounding "No."

One Size Doesn't Fit all with Fluoride

One interesting tidbit about fluoride is that it is the only thing added to our drinking water that is there to treat the person drinking the water. Chlorine is added to the water to treat the water. Fluoride is added to the water to treat the person.

How would you feel about the government deciding that we were all much too cranky, so they put anti-depressants in the water supply. We wouldn't stand for it, for many reasons! Not everyone needs those anti-depressants, and some people are already on them. There are undesirable side effects with anti-depressants. Some people are opposed to medication entirely. These medications don't work on everyone's depression, even if everyone were depressed. And lastly, why in the world would it be appropriate for a child to have the same dose of that medication as an adult?

Those exact same arguments apply for fluoride. We are all being medicated with fluoride through our drinking water. And usually, we are being over-medicated, even if you believe that fluoride is a valid "medication" (I don't, and I don't provide it in my practice). Let's talk about a hypothetical young child living in an area where the water is fluoridated.

The parents are very diligent, and want to make sure their child is getting enough fluoride. The pediatrician recommends a fluoride supplement, without finding out if they have fluoridated water. Wanting the best for their child, they give him the supplement every day. When it's time to brush teeth, they use a typical fluoride toothpaste—bubblegum, so the child makes sure to swallow some of that yummy stuff. Then he wants to use mommy's mouth rinse that contains fluoride, so she gives him some to rinse with, not worrying if he swallows a little. Every cup of water, drink of fruit juice, and most processed foods have additional fluoride in them. The pediatrician wasn't negligent in prescribing the supplement, but didn't take into account the fact that fluoride was already coming from many sources. The child has now been overdosed with fluoride through common and recommended products and practices.

When Should You Use Fluoride?

With all this negative talk about fluoride, it would seem there is no reason to ever use it. I wouldn't entirely agree with that. It is a mineral that can help remineralize teeth, if used directly on the tooth. I do occasionally advocate topical use of fluoride, directly on the tooth, and only exactly where it is needed. There is never a reason to take fluoride internally, but topically it can be effective to stop progression of an early cavity if used for a limited time and very carefully.

If you live in an area with water fluoridation, I highly recommend a type of water filter like the Berkey Filtration System with added fluoride filters. It can effectively filter out fluoride. You can also use a Reverse Osmosis water system or a Water Alkalizer or Ionizer, but there are dental concerns with both. If you use a Reverse Osmosis system, you must remineralize the water by adding minerals, or the water will steal minerals from your teeth. With the Water Alkalizer you cannot drink the water with meals or it will interfere with stomach acid and you will not absorb needed nutrients from your food. Be careful and thoughtful about your water and what is in it to ensure the best health for you and your family.

Chapter Eleven: Improve Your Smile

I'm going to finish with something a little less serious, and a lot more fun! There have been countless studies that show the effect a great smile can have on your confidence, which leads to other success. I spent the first half of my career focused on creating new smiles, and it is always so rewarding to change a life. As I have transitioned to a more holistic practice, I have come up with natural, more conservative methods to improve your smile.

My mantra is *"Clean the Outside, Nourish the Inside".* What this means is that whiteness comes from the outside and the inside, and you can improve both. If you have stains on your teeth, you can remove them with a simple whitening paste.

> **Tooth-Whitening Paste**
> 1 part Baking soda
> 1 part Sea Salt
>
> *Mix with water to make a paste. Apply with a toothbrush in circular motions to remove stains a couple of times a week. Do after your regular brushing.*

Oil Pulling

Deeper stains can be pulled out with Oil Pulling. Oil pulling is an ancient Indian practice that involves swishing oil in your mouth to remove bacteria and lead to better dental health. Does it work or is it just a folk remedy? Research has shown there are beneficial effects of oil pulling, including:

- Oil pulling can kill bacteria that cause tooth decay. Some alternative medicine practitioners also claim that it can help treat several diseases.[1]
- It moisturizes gums and increases saliva production, which can reduce bacteria.[2]
- Can naturally reduce inflammation and bacteria.[2]
- Significantly reduces the number of harmful bacteria found in the saliva and plaque.[3]
- Causes a significant decrease in bad breath.[4]
- Reduces plaque and improves gum health.[5]

> **How to Do Oil Pulling in 4 Simple Steps**
> 1. Measure one tablespoon of oil, such as coconut, sesame or olive oil.
> 2. Swish it around in your mouth for 15-20 minutes, being careful not to swallow any.
> 3. Spit the oil into a trash can once you're done. Avoid spitting it into the sink or toilet, as this can cause a buildup of oil, which may lead to clogging.
> 4. Rinse your mouth well with water before eating or drinking anything.
>
> *Repeat these steps a few times per week or daily as you find what works for your schedule. You can start with 5 minutes of swishing working up to 15-20 minutes per time. Best results come when doing it first thing in the morning on an empty stomach.*

Natural Whitening

If your teeth are darker then you would like, you can nourish them from the inside. Remember to get enough Fat Soluble Vitamins from the suggestions in Chapter Five.

Professional whitening

If you've tried everything here and you are not having any success, professional whitening may be necessary to get your teeth as white as you would like. Professional whitening systems all use either hydrogen or carbamide peroxide. These products do change those enamel crystals, but as long as you have enough nutrients, minerals and vitamins in your system, you will be able to remineralize the tooth.

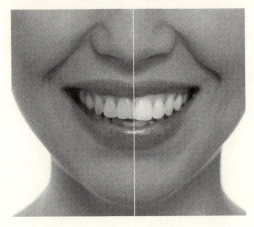

One caution is that if mercury fillings are in the mouth, these whitening peroxides will cause more mercury to be released. So, I do not recommend tooth whitening with peroxides until all the mercury is removed from the teeth.

Porcelain or resin veneers

In our office we provide ultra tooth-conserving cosmetic restorations. For long-lasting changes, we recommend Durathin veneers from Experience Dental Labs. These differ from regular veneers in that no tooth structure has to be removed to place them. We can change the shape, size and color of your tooth without damaging the tooth at all. These are not possible for every smile and every tooth, so ask your Holistic dentist if you are a candidate for Durathins.

For a less expensive, shorter term solution, we have also pioneered *BioLuxe Resin* veneers. These are custom veneers made out of dental resin. They also are very thin and require little to no tooth structure be removed to place them. The advantage is that they can be constructed at the dental chair and don't require a second visit. The disadvantage is that they will pick up stain over time and may need to be replaced for cosmetic reasons in five to ten years after placement.

Both type of veneers are conservative and beautiful. They will transform a smile overnight!

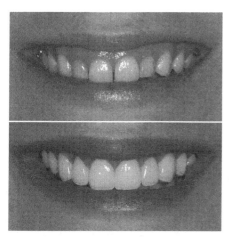
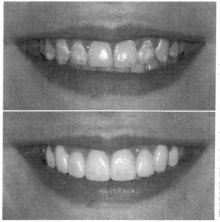

Photos and dentistry by Dr. Chase Larsen, DMD at Total Care Dental

In Conclusion

I hope you have enjoyed reading this book and learning more about how to keep your mouth and your body healthy. There is so much information out there. It is difficult to sift through all of it and determine what is best for you and your family. My intent was to help you do that, and to learn key information you can share with others. You CAN have a healthy mouth for life. It's not secret, magic or difficult. Now you have the tools to make that happen.

If you would like more information, go to my website:

www.totalcaredental.com. I update it weekly.

Remember, it is your mouth and your body. Take care of yourself and use this information to find a holistic dentist that can help you with that care. To your health!

Quick-Start Guide to Holistic Dental Care

Toothbrush:
- Bass soft-bristle toothbrush –Amazon.com
- Oral B Electric Toothbrush –Amazon.com

Toothpaste:
- Earthpaste–www.earthpaste.com
- Betonite Clay–Amazon.com

Tongue Cleaners:
- Oolit tongue scraper
- BreathRX –Amazon.com

Clean Between Aids:
- Water Pik –Amazon.com
- Shower Flosser –www.showerfloss.com
- Go Betweens –Amazon.com

Mouthrinse
- Tooth and Gum Tonic –Amazon.com

Cod Liver Oil Supplements:
- Extra Virgin – Rosita from corganic.com
- Fermented– Green Pastures from Amazon.com or codliveroilshop.com

Butter
- Kerrygold Butter – grocery and health food stores
- Butter oil –Amazon.com
- Ghee – Amazon.com or grocery stores

Dirty Dozen and Clean 15 list for shopping
- www.ewg.org/foodnews/clean-fifteen.php

Oral Probiotics
- Florassist –lifeextension.com

Resources

Where to find a Holistic Dentist

Dr. Tom McGuire's Mercury Safe Dentist Directory
www.dentalwellness4u.com/freeservices/find_dentists.html

Insider's Guide to Holistic Dentists
www.greensmoothiegirl.com/healthymouth/getlist/

International Academy of Oral Medicine and Toxicology (IAOMT)
www.iaomt.org

Organizations for More Information

International Academy of Biological Dentistry and Medicine
www.iabdm.org

Holistic Dental Association
www.holisticdental.org

Academy of Biomimetic Dentistry
www.aobmd.org

Educational Resources

Citizens for Safe Drinking Water
www.nofluoride.com

Fluoride Action Network
www.fluoridealert.org

Price-Pottenger Foundation
www.ppnf.org

Alternative Services

Dental Materials Compatibility Testing- Clifford Consulting and Research, Inc.
www.ccrlab.com

Hair and Tissue Mineral Analysis – Analytical Research Laboratories, Inc.
www.arltma.com

Hair and Tissue Mineral Analysis- Doctor's Data, Inc.
www.doctorsdata.com

Bioelectrical devices – Synergy Health Systems
www.synergyhealthsystems.com

**Whole-Body Wellness –
Total Care Dental and Dr. Michelle Jorgensen's updates**
www.totalcaredental.com

Suggested Reading

Alexander, Leslie M. PhD, and Straub-Bruce, Linda A, RDH. Dental Herbalism: *Natural Therapies For The Mouth*. Rochester, VT: Healing Arts Press, 2014.

Altman, Nathaniel. *The New Oxygen Prescription: The Miracle of Oxidative Therapies*. Rochester, Vermont: Healing Arts Press, 2017.

Becker, Robert O., MD and Seldon, Gary. *The Body Electric: Electromagnetism and The Foundation of Life*. New York: William Morrow and Company, Inc. 1985.

Breiner, Mark A, DDS. *Whole-Body Dentistry: A Complete Guide To Understanding The Impact Of Dentistry On Total Health*. Fairfield, CT: Quantum Health Press, 2011.

Chi, Tsu-Tsair, NMD, PhD. *Dr. Chi's Fingernail And Tongue Analysis*. Anaheim, CA: Chi's Enterprise, 2010.

Fallon, Sally, and Enig, Mary G, PhD. *Nourishing Traditions: The Cookbook That Challenges Politically Correct Nutrition And The Diet Dictocrats*. Washington DC: NewTrends Publishing, 2001.

Galland, Leo, MD. *The Four Pillars of Healing*. New York: Random House, 1997.

Gittleman, Ann Louise. *Zapped: Why Your Cell Phone Shouldn't Be Your Cell Phone And 1,268 Ways To Outsmart The Hazards Of Electronic Pollution*. New York, NY: Harper Collins, 2011.

Gundry, Steven R. MD. *The Plant Paradox*. New York: Harper Wave, 2017.

Kahn, Sandra, and Ehrlich, Paul R. Jaws: *The Story Of A Hidden Epidemic*. Stanford, CA: Environmental Health Sciences Book, 2018.

Katz, Sando Ellix. *Wild Fermentation: The Flavor, Nutrition And Craft Of Live-Culture Foods.* White River Junction, Vermont: Chelsea Green Publishing, 2003.

Levy, Thomas E, MD, JD. *Hidden Epidemic: Silent Oral Infections Cause Most Heart Attacks And Breast Cancers.* Henderson, NV: Medfox, 2017.

Meining, George, DDS. *Root Canal Cover-up.* Ojai, CA: Bion Publishing, 1994.

Morse, Robert, ND. *The Detox Miracle Sourcebook: Raw Foods And Herbs For Complete Cellular Regeneration.* Chino Valley, AZ: Kalindi Press, 2004.

Nuzum, Dan, ND and Nuzum-Orozco, Gina. *Detox For Life: How To Minimize Toxins And Maximize Your Body's Ability To Heal.* USA: Tru Publishing, 2017.

Openshaw, Robyn. Vibe: *Unlock The Energetic Frequencies Of Limitless Health, Love And Success.* New York: North Star Way, 2017.

Price, Weston, DDS. *Nutrition and Physical Degeneration.* Lemon Grove, CA: Price-Pottenger Nutrition Foundation, 1945.

Rau, Thomas, MD. *Biological Medicine: The Future of Natural Healing.* Germany: Semmelweis-Institut, 2016.

Tennant, Jerry MD, PSc. *Healing Is Voltage: The Handbook.* San Bernadino, CA: The Tennant Institute, 2013.

Urbanek, Karen, HHP. *Live With Outrageous Energy: Thrive Without Fear, Sickness And Disease!* West Bend, WI: Karen's Energy, 2014.

References

Yale University. n.d. "About Yale: Yale Facts." Accessed May 1, 2017. https://www.yale.edu/about-yale/yale-facts.

Chapter One

1. Levy, Thomas E. 2017. *Hidden Epidemic: Silent Oral Infections Cause Most Heart Attacks and Breast Cancers.* Henderson: MedFox Publishing.

2. Breiner, Mark. 2011. *Whole-Body Dentistry: A Complete Guide to Understanding the Impact of Dentistry on Total Health.* Fairfield: Quantum Health Press.

Chapter Two

1. Encyclopedia Britannica. 2018. *Tooth Anatomy.* https://www.britannica.com/science/tooth-anatomy

Chapter Three

1. Centers for Disease Control and Prevention. 2016. *Hygiene Related Diseases.* https://www.cdc.gov/healthywater/hygiene/disease/dental_caries.html#one

2. Dye BA, Tan S, Smith V, Lewis BG, Barker LK, Thornton-Evans G, Eke PI, Beltrán-Aguilar ED, Horowitz AM, Li CH. *Trends in oral health status, United States, 1988-1994 and 1999-2004.* Vital Health Stat 11. 2007;(248):1-92.

3. American Dental Association Health Policy Institute. 2017. *US Dental Expenditures.* https://www.ada.org/~/media/ADA/Science%20and%20Research/HPI/Files/HPIBrief_1217_1.pdf?la=en

4. Larmas, M. Journal of Dental Research. *Dental Caries Seen from the Pulpal Side: a Nontraditional Approach.* 2003; 82(4):253-256.

5. Shklar, G; Carranza, FA: *The Historical Background of Periodontology.* In Newman, MG; Takei, HH; Carrana FA, editors: Carranza's Clinical Periodontology, 9th Edition. Philadelphia: W.B. Saunders Company, 2002. page 8.

6. Price, WA. *Nutrition and Physical Degeneration.* California, 2003. Price-Pottenger Nutrition Foundation.

7. Page, ME. *Degeneration Regeneration.* 1949. Biochemical Research Foundation.

8. Roggenkamp C, Leonora J. *Dentinal Fluid Transport.* 2005. Loma Linda University Press.

9. Statovci, D., Aguilera, M., MacSharry, J., & Melgar, S. (2017). *The Impact of Western Diet and Nutrients on the Microbiota and Immune Response at Mucosal Interfaces.* Frontiers in immunology, 8, 838. doi:10.3389/fimmu.2017.00838

Chapter Four

1. Huynh NC-N, Everts V, Leethanakul C, Pavasant P, Ampornaramveth RS (2016) *Rinsing with Saline Promotes Human Gingival Fibroblast Wound Healing In Vitro.* PLoS ONE 11(7): e0159843.

2. Mercola J. *Toxic Toothpaste Ingredients You Need to Avoid.* 2015. https://articles.mercola.com/sites/articles/archive/2015/09/09/toxic-toothpaste-ingredients.aspx

3. Colgate Professional. *Taking Care of Your Teeth.* 2007. https://www.colgateprofessional.com/education/patient-education/topics/oral-hygiene-basics/taking-care-of-your-teeth

4. Mark AM. Journal of the American Dental Association. *Limiting the Effects of Dry Mouth.* 2017. https://jada.ada.org/article/S0002-8177(17)30467-1/pdf

Chapter Five

1. Price, WA. *Nutrition and Physical Degeneration.* La Mesa: Price-Pottenger Nutrition Foundation. 2004.

2. Op. cit. p 441, 171, 174

3. Price, WA. Journal of the American Dental Association, 1936:888.

4. Price, WA. *"Field Studies among Some African Tribes on the Relation of their nutrition to the incidence of dental caries and dental arch deformities"* Journal of the American Dental Association. 23:888, May 1936.

5. Bier D, et al. (eds): *Nutrition for the Primary Care Provider.* World Rev Nutr Diet. Basel, Karger, 2015, vol 111, pp 38-44 (DOI:10.1159/000362295)

6. Fletcher J. Medical News Today. *"All you need to know about fat-soluble vitamins."* 2017. https://www.medicalnewstoday.com/articles/320310.php

7. Masterjohn C. The Weston A. Price Foundation. *"Nutritional Adjuncts to the Fat-Soluble Vitamins".* 2013. https://www.westonaprice.org/health-topics/abcs-of-nutrition/nutritional-adjuncts-to-the-fat-soluble-vitamins/

8. Lin S. *"Cod Liver Oil Ultimate Guide: Extra Virgin vs. Fermented".* Accessed November 17, 2018. https://www.drstevenlin.com/cod-liver-oil-extra-virgin-vs-fermented/

9. National Institutes of Health Office of Dietary Supplements. *"Vitamin D".* 2018. https://ods.od.nih.gov/factsheets/VitaminD-HealthProfessional/

10. Arnanson A. Healthline.com. *"Antioxidants explained in human terms."* 2017. https://www.healthline.com/nutrition/antioxidants-explained

11. Gunnars K. Healthline.com. *"Are vegetable and seed oils good for your health?"* 2018. https://www.healthline.com/nutrition/are-vegetable-and-seed-oils-bad

12. Proper Calcium Use: *Vitamin K2 as a Promoter of Bone and Cardiovascular Health.* Integr Med (Encinitas). 2015;14(1):34-9.

13. Schiffman R. Tale Environment 360. *"Why it's time to stop punishing our soils with fertilizers."* 2017. https://e360.yale.edu/features/why-its-time-to-stop-punishing-our-soils-with-fertilizers-and-chemicals

14. Mercola.com. *"The milk myth: What your body really needs."* 2009. https://articles.mercola.com/sites/articles/archive/2009/07/18/the-milk-myth-what-your-body-really-needs.aspx

15. Pollan M. Frontline PBS interview. Accessed on November 17, 2018. https://www.pbs.org/wgbh/pages/frontline/shows/meat/interviews/pollan.html

16. Real Milk Finder. Weston A Price Foundation. Accessed on November 17, 2018. https://www.realmilk.com/real-milk-finder/

17. Informed Health Online [Internet]. Cologne, Germany: Institute for Quality and Efficiency in Health Care (IQWiG); 2006-. *Causes and diagnosis of lactose intolerance.* 2010 Sep 15 [Updated 2015 Jun 17]. https://www.ncbi.nlm.nih.gov/books/NBK310263/

18. Mozaffarian D: *Changes in diet and lifestyle and long-term weight gain in women and men.* N Engl J Med 2011, 364:2392-2404.

19. Chen M, Sun Q, Giovannucci E, Mozaffarian D, Manson JE, Willett WC, Hu FB: *Dairy consumption and risk of type 2 diabetes: 3 cohorts of US adults and an updated meta- analysis.* BMC Med 2014 http://dx.doi.org/10.1186/s12916-014-0215-1.

20. Eussen SJPM, van Dongen MCJM, Wijckmans N, den Biggelaar L, Oude Elferink SJWH, Singh-Povel CM, Schram MT, Sep SJS, van der Kallen CJ, Koster A et al.: *Consumption of dairy foods in relation to impaired glucose metabolism and type 2 diabetes mellitus: the Maastricht Study.* Br J Nutr 2016, 115:1453-1461.

21. Soedamah-Muthu SS, Masset G, Verberne L, Geleijnse JM, Brunner EJ: *Consumption of dairy products and associations with incident diabetes, CHD and mortality in the Whitehall II study.* Br J Nutr 2013, 109:718-726.

22. Tapsell LC: *Fermented dairy food and CVD risk.* Br J Nutr 2015, 113:131-135.

23. Iwasa M, Aoi W, Mune K, Yamauchi H, Furuta K, Sasaki S, Takeda K, Harada K, Wada S, Nakamura Y et al.: *Fermented milk improves glucose metabolism in exercise-induced muscle damage in young healthy men.* Nutr J 2013 https://nutritionj.biomedcentral.com/articles/10.1186/1475-2891-12-83

24. An SY, Lee MS, Jeon JY, Ha ES, Kim TH, Yoon JY, Ok CO, Lee HK, Hwang WS, Choe SJ et al.: *Beneficial effects of fresh and fermented kimchi in prediabetic individuals.* Ann Nutr Metab 2013, 63:111-119.

25. Lorea Baroja M, Kirjavainen PV, Hekmat S, Reid G: *Anti-inflammatory effects of probiotic yogurt in inflammatory bowel disease patients.* Clin Exp Immunol 2007, 149:470-479.

26. Tillisch K, Labus J, Kilpatrick L, Jiang Z, Stains J, Ebrat B, Guyonnet D, Legrain-Raspaud S, Trotin B, Naliboff BME: *Consumption of fermented milk product with probiotics modulates brain activity.* Gastroenterology 2014 http://dx.doi.org/10.1053/j.gastro.2013.02.043

27. Hilimire MR, DeVylder JE, Forestell CA: *Fermented foods, neuroticism, and social anxiety: an interaction model.* Psychiatry Res 2015, 228:203-208.

28. Omagari K, Sakaki M, Tsujimoto Y, Shiogama Y, Iwanaga A, Ishimoto M, Yamaguchi A, Masuzumi M, Kawase M, Ichimura M et al.: *Coffee consumption is inversely associated with depressive status in Japanese patients with type 2 diabetes.* J Clin Biochem Nutr 2014, 55:135-142.

29. National Osteoporosis Foundation. *A guide to Calcium Rich Foods.* Accessed on November 17, 2018. https://www.nof.org/patients/treatment/calciumvitamin-d/a-guide-to-calcium-rich-foods/

30. Whittamore JM, Hatch M. *The role of intestinal oxalate transport in hyperoxaluria and the formation of kidney stones in animals and man.* Urolithiasis. 2016;45(1):89-108.

31. Harvard health Publishing. *"What's the scoop on bone broth?"* 2015. https://www.health.harvard.edu/healthy-eating/whats-the-scoop-on-bone-soup

32. AlgaeCal. *The Dangers of Sugar and Bone Health: More Addictive Than Cocaine?"* 2014. https://www.algaecal.com/expert-insights/dangers-sugar-bone-health-addictive-cocaine/

33. Page ME, Abrams HL. *Health vs. Disease, a Revolution in medical Thinking.* St. Petersburg, Florida: Page Foundation, 1096. 57

34. Nagel R. *Cure Tooth Decay.* Oregon: Golden Child Publishing. 2012.

35. Tannenbaum and others. *Vitamins and Minerals, in Food Chemistry*, 2nd edition. OR Fennema, ed. Marcel Dekker, Inc., New York, 1985, p 445.

36. Johansen K and others. *Degradation of phytate in soaked diets for pigs.* Department of Animal Health, Welfare and Nutrition, Danish Institute of Agricultural Sciences, Research Centre Foulum, Tjele, Denmark.

37. Navert B and Sandstrom B. *Reduction of the phytate content of bran by leavening in bread and its effect on zinc absorption in man.* British Journal of Nutrition 1985 53:47-53; Phytic acid added to white-wheat bread inhibits fractional apparent magnesium absorption in humans 1-3. Bohn T and others. American Journal of Clinical Nutrition. 2004 79:418-23.

38. Srivastava BN and others. *Influence of Fertilizers and Manures on the Content of Phytin and Other Forms of Phosphorus in Wheat and Their Relation to Soil Phosphorus.* Journal of the Indian Society of Soil Science. 1955 III:33-40.

39. Reddy NR and others. *Food Phytates*, CRC Press, 2001.

40. Figures collected from various sources. *Inhibitory effect of nuts on iron absoprtion.* American Journal of Clinical Nutrition 1988 47:270-4; J Anal At Spectrum. 2004 19,1330-1334; Journal of Agriculture and Food Chemistry 1994, 42:2204-2209.

41. *Effects of soaking, germination and fermentation on phytic acid, total and in vitro soluble zinc in brown rice.* Food Chemistry 2008 110:821-828.

42. Wills MR and others. *Phytic Acid and Nutritional Rickets in Immigrants.* The Lancet, April 8, 1972, 771-773.

43. Walker ARP and others. *The Effect of Bread Rich in Phytate Phosphorus on the metabolism of Certain Mineral Salts with Special Reference to Calcium.* The Biochemical Journal 1948 42(1):452-461.

44. *Iron absorption in man: ascorbic acid and dose-depended inhibition.* American Journal of Clinical Nutrition. Jan 1989 49(1):140-144

45. *Inhibitory effect of nuts on iron absorption.* American Journal of Clinical Nutrition 1988 47:270-4.

46. Reddy NR and others. *Food Phytates*, CRC Press, 2001.

47. Vucenik I and Shamsuddin AM. *Cancer inhibition by inositol hexaphosphate (IP6) and inositol: from laboratory to clinic.* The Journal of Nutrition 2003 Nov 133(11 Suppl 1); Jenab M and Thompson LU (August 2000). *Phytic acid in wheat bran affects colon morphology, cell differentiation and apoptosis.* Carcinogenesis 2000 Aug 21(8):1547-52.

48. Egli I and others. *The Influence of Soaking and Germination on the Phytase Activity and Phytic Acid Content of Grains and Seeds Potentially Useful for Complementary Feeding.* Journal of Food Science 2002 Vol. 67, Nr. 9.

49. The Nourishing Home. *"How to Soak Grains for Optimal Nutrition".* Accessed on November 17, 2018. https://thenourishinghome.com/2012/03/how-to-soak-grains-for-optimal-nutrition/

50. Cottis H. Whole Lifestyle Nutrition. *"Are Soaking Grains And Legumes Necessay And How To Properly Soak And Prepare Them."* Accessed on November 17, 2018. https://wholelifestylenutrition.com/health/is-soaking-grains-and-legumes-necessary-and-how-to-properly-soak-and-prepare-them/

51. Mariani-Costantini R, Mariani-Costantini A. *An outline of the history of pellagra in Italy.* J Anthropol Sci. 2007;85:163-171

52. Ginnaio M. *Pellagra in Late Nineteenth Century Italy: Effects of a Deficiency Disease.* Popul (english Ed.) 2011.

53. Gentilcore D. *Peasants & Pellagra in 19th-century Italy.* Hist Today. 2014

54. Hegyi J, Schwartz RA, Hegyi V. *Pellagra: Dermatitis, dementia, and diarrhea.* International Journal of Dermatology. 2004.

55. Lanska D. *Historical aspects of the major neurological vitamin deficiency disorders: the water-soluble B vitamins.* Handb Clin Neurol. 2009.

56. Bollet AJ. *Politics and pellagra: The epidemic of pellagra in the U.S. in the early twentieth century.* Yale J Biol Med. 1992.

57. Elmore JG, Feinstein AR. *Joseph Goldberger: An unsung hero of American clinical epidemiology.* Ann Intern Med. 1994.

58. Hotz C and others. *A home-based method to reduce phytate content and increase zinc bioavailability in maize based complementary diets.* International Journal of Food Science and Nutrition 2001 52:133–42.

Chapter Six

1. American Association of Endodontists. *American Dental Association Survey of Dental Services Rendered.* 2007. https://www.aae.org/specialty/about-aae/news-room/endodontic-treatment-statistics/

2. Tabassum S, Khan FR. *Failure of endodontic treatment: The usual suspects.* Eur J Dent. 2016;10(1):144-7.

3. Lin LM, Pascon EA, Skribner J, Gängler P, Langeland K. *Clinical, radiographic, and histologic study of endodontic treatment failures.* Oral Surg Oral Med Oral Pathol. 1991;71:603–11.

4. Endo MS, Ferraz CC, Zaia AA, Almeida JF, Gomes BP. *Quantitative and qualitative analysis of microorganisms in root-filled teeth with persistent infection: Monitoring of the endodontic retreatment.* Eur J Dent. 2013;7:302–9

5. Hoen MM, Pink FE. *Contemporary endodontic retreatments: An analysis based on clinical treatment findings.* J Endod. 2002;28:834–6.

6. Lin LM, Skribner JE, Gaengler P. *Factors associated with endodontic treatment failures.* J Endod. 1992;18:625–7.

7. Ray HA, Trope M. *Periapical status of endodontically treated teeth in relation to the technical quality of the root filling and the coronal restoration.* Int Endod J. 1995;28:12–8.

8. Crump MC, Natkin E. *Relationship of broken root canal instruments to endodontic case prognosis: A clinical investigation.* J Am Dent Assoc. 1970;80:1341–7.

9. Wolcott J, Ishley D, Kennedy W, Johnson S, Minnich S, Meyers J. *A 5 yr clinical investigation of second mesiobuccal canals in endodontically treated and retreated maxillary molars.* J Endod. 2005;31:262–4.

10. Lemagner f, Maret D, Peters O, et al. (2015) *Prevalence of apical bone defects and evaluation of associated factors detected with cone=beam computed tomographic images.* Journal of Endodontics, 41:1043-1047.

11. Price, WA, *Dental Infections, Oral and Systemic, Vol. I*, Penton Pub Co. Ohio, USA, 1923.

12 Pessi T1, Karhunen V, Karjalainen PP, et al. *"Bacterial signatures in thrombus aspirates of patients with myocardial infarction."* Circulation. 2013 Mar 19;127(11):1219-28, e1-6. doi: 10.1161/CIRCULATIONAHA.112.001254. Epub 2013 Feb 15.

13. Aarabi G, Schnabel RB, Heydecke G, Seedorf U. *Potential Impact of Oral Inflammations on Cardiac Functions and Atrial Fibrillation.* Biomolecules. 2018;8(3):66. Published 2018 Aug 1. doi:10.3390/biom8030066

14. Wilson K, Liu Z, Huang J, Roosaar A, Axéll T, Ye W. *Poor oral health and risk of incident myocardial infarction: A prospective cohort study of Swedish adults, 1973-2012.* Sci Rep. 2018;8(1):11479. Published 2018 Jul 31. doi:10.1038/s41598-018-29697-9

15. Pessi T, Viiri LE, Raitoharju E, et al. *Interleukin-6 and microRNA profiles induced by oral bacteria in human atheroma derived and healthy smooth muscle cells.* Springerplus. 2015;4:206. Published 2015 Apr 30. doi:10.1186/s40064-015-0993-8

16. Thomas S, Ghosh J, Porter J, Cockcroft A, Rautemaa-Richardson R. *Periodontal disease and late-onset aortic prosthetic vascular graft infection.* Case Rep Vasc Med. 2015;2015:768935.

17. Louhelainen AM, Aho J, Tuomisto S, et al. *Oral bacterial DNA findings in pericardial fluid.* J Oral Microbiol. 2014;6:25835. Published 2014 Nov 19. doi:10.3402/jom.v6.25835

18. *Ozone therapy in dentistry: A strategic review.* J Nat Sci Biol Med. 2011;2(2):151-3.

19. *Probiotics and oral health.* Eur J Dent. 2010;4(3):348-55.

20. *Galvanism in the Oral Cavity.* Journal of the American Dental Association. 1940; 27(9): 1471–1475

21. Levy TE. *Hidden Epidemic: Silent Oral Infection Cause Most Heart Attacks and Breast Cancers.* 2017; Nevada- MedFox Publishing.

22. Bouquot JE, LaMarche MG. *Ischemic Osteonecrosis under fixed partial denture pntics: Radiograph and microscopic features in 38 patinets with chronic pain.* J Prosthetic Dentistry. 1999; 81:148-158. https://www.sciencedirect.com/science/article/pii/S0022391399702428

23. Barrett WC: *Oral Pathology and Practice.* Philadelphia, PA. SS White Dental Mfg. Co 1898.

24. Noel HR: *A lecture on caries and necrosis of the bone.* Am J Dent Sci (series 3): 189, 1868.

25. Black GV: *A work on special dental pathology.* Chicago: Medico-Dental Co, 1915; 388-391.

26. Neville BW, Damm DD, Allen CM, Bouquot JE. *Oral and Maxillofacial Pathology.* Philadelphia: WB Saunders Co; 2009. 866-869.

27. Hailey B. *Characterization and identification of chemical toxicants isolated from cavitational material and infected root canalled teeth; in situ testing of teeth for toxicity and infection.* Proceedings of Annual meeting, International Academy of Oral Medicine and Toxicology; San Diego, California; 1997.

28. Shankland WE. *Medullary and odontogenic disease in the painful jaw: clinical pathologic review of 500 consecutive lesions.* Cranio. 12002 Oct; 20(4): 295-303.

29. Ratner EJ, Person P, Kleinman DJ, Shklar G, Socransky SS: *Jawbone cavities and trigeminal and atypical facial neuralgias.* Oral Surg 1970, 48, no.1: 3-20

30. Bouquot JE, Roberts AM, Person P: *Neuralgia-inducing cavitational osteonecrosis (NICO):Osteomyelitis in 224 jawbone samples from patients with facial neuralgias.* Oral Surg Oral Med Oral Pathol 1992; 73: 312-315

31. Lechner J, von Baehr V. *Rantes and fibroblast growth factor 2 in jaw bone cavitations: triggers for systemic disease?* Int J Gen Med. 6 (2013): 277-290

32. *The Cancer/Cavitation Connection,* North Carolina Institute of Technology, http://www.cancercured.org/gpage6.html

33. *Bacteria recovered from teeth with apical periodontitis after antimicrobial endodontic treatment.* Chavez de Paz LE, Dahlen G, Molander A, Moller A, Bergenholtz G. Int Endod J. 2003 Jul;36(7):500-8.

34. *Jawbone cavities and trigeminal and atypical facial neuralgias,* Ratner DJ et al, Oral Surg. Oral Med Oral Pathol, 1979, 48(1):3-20.

35. *Osteocavitation lesions: a case report,* Shankland, WE, Cranio,1993, 11(3):232-236.

36. *Unhealed extraction sites mimicking TMJ pain,* Dupont JD, Gen Dent 2000, 48(1): 82-85.

37. *Bone Cavities, Trigeminal Neuralgia, Atypical Facial Pain,* Robert E Mc Mahon DDS. www.dentistryhealth.ocm/pathology.html

38. *Mouth Infections and the Relation to Systemic Diseases, Vol I and II,* Malcolm Graeme MacNevin, MD, F.A.C.P; Harold Sterns Vaughn, M.C. DACS www.dentistryhealth.ocm/pathology.html

39. *"EPA Memorandum of Understanding on Reducing Dnetal Amalgam Discharges."* Dental Effluent Guidelines. Environmental Protection Agency. Web. 2016

40. Brown EH, Hansen RT. *The Key to Ultimate Health.* Fullerton; Advanced Health Research Publishing: 1998:32-33.

41. Ring ME (2005). *Founders of a profession: the original subscribers to the first dental journal in the world.* The Journals of the American college of Dentist 72 (2): 20-5.

42. Legal brief filed in 1995 by attorneys for the ADA in WH Tolhurst vs. Johnson and Johnson Consumer Products, Inc; Engelhard Corporation; ABE Dental Inc; The American Dental Association, et al in the Superior Court of the State of California, in and for the county of Santa Clara, CA. Case No. 718228.

43. Aschner M, Aschner JL. *Mercury neurotoxocity: mechanisms of blood-brain narrier transport.* Neuroscience Biobehav Rev. 1990; 14(2): 169-76.

44. IAOMT. *Learning Aid Mercury 102.* Accessed on November 17, 2018. https://iaomt.org/wp-content/uploads/02_course_documents.pdf

45. *Smoking Teeth = Poison Gas.* https://www.youtube.com/watch?v=h-qIdGwAMxxs

46. American Dental Association News Release. *American Dental Association Reaffirms Position on Dental Amalgam.* September 30, 2016.

47. Ministry of the Environment, Norway. *Minister of the Environment and International Development Erik Solheim: Bans mercury in products* [Press release]. 2007 December 21. Available from Government of Norway Web site: https://www.regjeringen.no/en/aktuelt/Bans-mercury-in-products/id495138/. Accessed December 15, 2015.

48. Swedish Chemicals Agency. *The Swedish Chemicals Agency's chemical products and biotechnical organisms regulations.* (KIFS 2008: 2 in English, consolidated up to KIFS 2012: 3). 2008: 29-30.

49. BIO Intelligence Service. *Study on the potential for reducing mercury pollution from dental amalgam and batteries.* Final Report prepared for the European Commission- DG ENV. 2012. Page 188. Available from the European Commission Web site: http://ec.europa.eu/environment/chemicals/mercury/pdf/final_report_110712.pdf. Accessed December 15, 2015.

50. BIO Intelligence Service. *Study on the potential for reducing mercury pollution from dental amalgam and batteries.* Final Report prepared for the European Commission- DG ENV. 2012. Page 40. Available from the European Commission Web site: http://ec.europa.eu/environment/chemicals/mercury/pdf/final_report_110712.pdf. Accessed December 15, 2015.

51. Health and Environment Alliance and Health Care without Harm. *Mercury and dental amalgams* [fact sheet]. 2007. Page 3. Available from Health and Environment Alliance Web site: http://www.env-health.org/IMG/pdf/HEA_009-07.pdf. Accessed December 15, 2015.

52. World Health Organization. *Mercury in Health Care:* Policy Paper. Geneva, Switzerland; August 2005: 1. Available from: http://www.who.int/water_sanitation_health/medicalwaste/mercurypolpaper.pdf. Accessed December 22, 2015.

53. International Acedemy of Oral Medicine and Toxicology (IOAMT). *Position Paper against Dental Mercury Amalgam Fillings for Medical and Dental Practitioners, Dental Students, Dental Patients, and Policy Makers.* Originally Released on April 16, 2013; Updated on March 2, 2016 Compiled, Developed, Released, and Updated by The IAOMT Scientific Review and Clinical Practice Guideline Committee: John Kall, DMD, FAGD, MIAOMT, Kindal Robertson, DDS, AIAOMT, Phillip Sukel, DDS, MIAOMT, Amanda Just, MS.

54. World Health Organization. *Mercury in Health Care* [policy paper]. August 2005: 1. Available from WHO Web site: http://www.who.int/water_sanitation_health/medicalwaste/mercurypolpaper.pdf. Accessed December 15, 2015.

55. Health Canada. *The Safety of Dental Amalgam*. 1996: 8, 13. Available from Health Canada Web site: http://www.hc-sc.gc.ca/dhp-mps/alt_formats/hpfb-dgpsa/pdf/md-im/dent_amalgam-eng.pdf. Accessed December 15, 2015.

56. IAOMT *Safe Mercury Amalgam Removal Technique (SMART)*. Accessed on November 17, 2018. https://iaomt.org/resources/safe-removal-amalgam-fillings/

57. Hodges RE, Minich DM. *Modulation of Metabolic Detoxification Pathways Using Foods and Food-Derived Components: A Scientific Review with Clinical Application.* J Nutr Metab. 2015;2015:760689.

Chapter Seven

1. Goswami S. *Biomimetic dentistry.* J Oral Res Rev 2018;10:28-32.

2. Ali, Afzal & Saraf, Prahlad & Patil, Jayaprakash & Gokani, Bhakti. (2017). *Biomimetic Materials in Dentistry.* Research & Reviews: Journal of Material Sciences. 05. 10.4172/2321-6212.1000188.

3. Gellar MC, Alter D. *The impact of Dentures on Nutritional Health of the Elderly.* The Journal of Aging Research and Clinical Practice. 2012.

4. Subhashini, M.H.R., Abirami, G., Jain, A.R. *Abutment selection in fixed partial denture–A review.* Drug Intervention Today. 2018; 10(1):111-115

5. Andreiotelli M, Wenz HJ, Kohal RJ. *Are ceramic implants a viable alternative to titanium implants? A systematic literature review.* Clin Oral Implants Res 2009;20 Suppl 4:32-47.

6. Schultze-Mosgau S, Schliephake H, Radespiel-Tröger M, Neukam FW. *Osseointegration of endodontic endosseous cones: Zirconium oxide vs titanium.* Oral Surg Oral Med Oral Pathol Oral Radiol Endod 2000;89:91-8.

7. Ideta, Takahiro & Yamazaki, Masaru & Kudou, Sadahiro & Higashida, Mitsuji & Mori, Shintarou & Kaneda, Takashi & Nakazawa, Masami. (2013). *Investigation of Radio Frequency Heating of Dental Implants Made of Titanium in 1.5 Tesla and 3.0 Tesla Magnetic Resonance Procedure: Measurement of the Temperature by Using Tissue-equivalent Phantom.* Nihon Hoshasen Gijutsu Gakkai zasshi. 69. 521-8. 10.6009/jjrt.2013_JSRT_69.5.521.

8. Care2.com. *32 Surprising sources of Toxic Heavy Metals.* Accessed on November 17, 2018. https://www.care2.com/greenliving/31-surprising-sources-of-toxic-heavy-metals.html

9. Blaschke C, Volz U. *Soft and hard tissue response to zirconium dioxide dental implants–A clinical study in man.* Neuro Endocrinol Lett 2006;27 Suppl 1:69-72.

10. Schultze-Mosgau S, Schliephake H, Radespiel-Tröger M, Neukam FW. *Osseointegration of endodontic endosseous cones: Zirconium oxide vs titanium.* Oral Surg Oral Med Oral Pathol Oral Radiol Endod 2000;89:91-8.

11. J Biomed Mater Res Part B 2009;519-9.

12. Lechner J, Noumbissi S, Baehr V. *Titanium implants and silent inflammation in jawbone—a critical interplay of dissolved titanium particles and cytokines TNF-α and RANTES/CCL5 on overall health?* EPMA Journal. 2018; 9(3):331-343.

Chapter Eight

1. Maxfield L, Crane JS. *Vitamin C Deficiency (Scurvy)* [Updated 2018 Aug 31]. In: StatPearls [Internet]. Treasure Island (FL): StatPearls Publishing; 2018 Jan-. Available from: https://www.ncbi.nlm.nih.gov/books/NBK493187/

2. American Academy of Periodontology. *CDC: Half of American Adults Have Periodontal Disease.* 2012. https://www.perio.org/consumer/cdc-study.htm

3. · Shangase SL, Mohangi GU, Hassam-Essa S, Wood NH (2013) *The association between periodontitis and systemic health: an overview.* SADJ 68: 8, 10-12.

4. *Gum Disease.* National Institute of Dental and Craniofacial Research. 2017. https://www.nidcr.nih.gov/sites/default/files/2017-09/periodontal-disease_0.pdf

5. Ahn J, Segers S, Hayes R (2012) *Periodontal disease, Porphyromonas gingivalis serum antibody levels and orodigestive cancer mortality.* Carcinogenesis 33: 1055-1058.

6. Michaud DS (2013) *Role of bacterial infections in pancreatic cancer.* Carcinogenesis 34: 2193-2197.

7. Whitmore SE, Lamont RJ (2014) *Oral bacteria and cancer.* PLoS Pathog 10: e1003933.

8. Yao CS, Waterfield JD, Shen Y, Haapasalo M, Macentee MI (2013) *In vitro antibacterial effect of carbamide peroxide on oral biofilm.* J Oral Microbiol 5.

9. Al-Katma MK, Bissada NF, Bordeaux JM, Sue J, Askari AD (2007) *Control of periodontal infection reduces the severity of active rheumatoid arthritis.* J Clin Rheumatol 13: 134-137.

10. Nasr SH, Radhakrishnan J, D'Agati VD (2013) *Bacterial infection-related glomerulonephritis in adults.* Kidney Int 83: 792-803.

11. Chukkapalli S, Rivera-Kweh MF, Velsko IM, Chen H, Zheng D, Bhattacharyya I, et al. (2015) *Chronic oral infection with major periodontal bacteria Tannerella forsythia modulates systemic atherosclerosis risk factors and inflammatory markers.* Pathogens and disease. 73.

12. Louhelainen AM, Aho J, Tuomisto S, Aittoniemi J, Vuento R, et al. (2014) *Oral bacterial DNA findings in pericardial fluid.* J Oral Microbiol 6: 25835.

13. Wahid A, Chaudhry S, Ehsan A, Butt S, Ali Khan A (2013) *Bidirectional Relationship between Chronic Kidney Disease and Periodontal Disease.* Pak J Med Sci 29: 211-215.

14. Noble JM, Scarmeas N, Papapanou PN (2013) *Poor oral health as a chronic, potentially modifiable dementia risk factor: review of the literature.* Curr Neurol Neurosci Rep 13: 384.

15. Dzingutė A, Pileičikienė G, Baltrušaitytė A, Skirbutis G. *Evaluation of the relationship between the occlusion parameters and symptoms of the temporomandibular joint disorder.* Acta Med Litu. 2017;24(3):167-175.

16. Oral Health Foundation. *Jaw Problems and Headaches.* Accessed November 17, 2018. https://www.dentalhealth.org/jaw-problems-and-headaches

Chapter Nine

1. Abou Neel EA, Aljabo A, Strange A, et al. *Demineralization-remineralization dynamics in teeth and bone.* Int J Nanomedicine. 2016;11:4743-4763. Published 2016 Sep 19. doi:10.2147/IJN.S107624

2. Reddy A, Norris DF, Momeni S, Waldo B, Ruby JD. *The pH of beverages in the United States.* Journal of the American Dental Association. 2016.

3. Institute of Medicine (US) Committee to Review Dietary Reference Intakes for Vitamin D and Calcium; Ross AC, Taylor CL, Yaktine AL, et al., editors. *Dietary Reference Intakes for Calcium and Vitamin D.* Washington (DC): National Academies Press (US); 2011. 2, Overview of Calcium. Available from: https://www.ncbi.nlm.nih.gov/books/NBK56060/

Chapter Ten

1. Kramer F. *Energetic Interrelations between Maxillo-Dental Region & Whole Organism. From Neural Therapy, Reflex Zones and Somatotopies: A Key to the Diagnostic and Therapeutic Understanding of Man's Ills*, a seminar guide compiled by the American Academy of Biological Dentistry, June 1989

2. Breiner MA. *Whole-Body Dentistry: A Complete Guide To Understanding The Impact Of Dentistry On Total Health.* Connecticut 2011. Quantum Health Press.

3. Ewing D. *Let the Tooth Be Known.* 1998. Holistic Health Alternatives.

4. Bale BF, Doneen AL, Vigerust DJ *High-risk periodontal pathogens contribute to the pathogenesis of atherosclerosis.* Postgrad Med J. 2017;93(1098)215-220. Published online 2016 doi: 10.1136/postgradmedj-2016-134279.

5. U.S. Department of Health and Human Services. *"HHS issues final recommendation for community water fluoridation."* Retrieved from http://www.hhs.gov/news/press/2015pres/04/20150427a.html

6. Mullenix, P.J., P.K. Denbesten, A. Schenior, and W.J. Kernan. *"Neurotoxicity of sodium fluoride in rats."* Neurotoxicology and Teratology 17.2 (March-April 1995): 169-177.

7. *"Scientist Who Spoke Out on Fluoride Ordered Reinstated to Job."* The Associated Press Feb. 11, 1994.

8. Cited as Radostits et al. 2000 (Radostits OM, Gay GC, Blood DC and Hinchcliff KW. 2000. Veterinary Medicine.9th edn. London, W B Saunders) in Swarup D, Dwivedi SK. *Environmental pollution and effects of lead and fluoride on animal health.* Indian Council of Agricultural Research Krishi Anusandhan Bhavan Pusa; New Delhi; 2002: Page 74.

9. National Research Council. *Fluoride in Drinking Water: A Scientific Review of EPA's Standards.* The National Academies Press: Washington, D.C. 2006. Page 44.

10. Sikora EJ, Chappelka AH. *Air Pollution Damage to Plants.* Alabama Cooperative Extension System. 2004.

11. National Research Council. *Fluoride in Drinking Water: A Scientific Review of EPA's Standards.* The National Academies Press: Washington, D.C. 2006. Page 44.

12. International Academy of Oral Medicine and Toxicology (IAOMT). *Position Paper against Fluoride Use in Water, Dental Materials, and Other Products for Dental and Medical Practitioners, Dental and Medical Students,Consumers, and Policy Makers.* Originally Released on September 22, 2017. Compiled, Developed, Written, and Released by Kennedy D, Just A, Kall J, Cole G.

13. Denbesten P, Li W. *Chronic fluoride toxicity: dental fluorosis.* Monogr Oral Sci. 2011;22:81-96.

https://www.hsph.harvard.edu/magazine/magazine_article/fluoridated-drinking-water/

https://www.cochrane.org/CD010856/ORAL_water-fluoridation-prevent-tooth-decay

Chapter Eleven

1. Singh A, Purohit B. *Tooth Brishing, oil pulling and tissue regeneration: A Review of holistic approaches to oral health.* Journal of Ayurveda and Integrative Medicine. 2011 Apr-June; 2(2):64-68

2. Shanbhag V. *Oil Pulling for maintaining oral hygiene–a review.* Journal of Traditional and Complementary Medicine. 2017 Jan; 7(1): 106-109.

3. Asokan S, Rathan J, Muthu MS, Rathna PV, Emmadi P, Raghuraman, Chanmundeswari. *Effect of oil pulling on Streptococcus mutans count in plaque and saliva using Dentocult SM Strip mutans test: a randomized, controlled, triple-blind study.* Journal of the Indian Society of Preventative Dentistry. 2008 Mar; 26(1): 12-7.

4. Asokan S, Kumar RS, Emmadi P, Raghuraman R, Sivakumar N. *Effect of oil pulling on halitosis and microorganisms causing halitosis: a randomized controlled pilot trial.* Journal of the Indian Society of Preventative Dentistry. 2011 Apr-June; 29(2): 90-4

5 Peedokayil FC, Sreenivasan P, Narayanan A. *Effect of Coconut oil in plaque related gingivitis–a preliminary report.* Nigerian Medical Journal. 2015 Mar-Apr; 56(2): 143-7.

Index

Acid 19, 20, 21, 23, 24, 26, 45, 49, 50-56, 60, 61, 68, 104, 111, 112-116, 122, 128

Acidogenic Theory 20

Acupuncture 5, 120

Alternative 3-6, 8, 10, 11, 12, 15, 36, 47, 49, 77, 83, 129, 134

Amalgam, Silver 2, 6, 73, 74-82

Bacteria 19, 20-25, 27-29, 32, 45, 49, 50, 61, 63-65, 67, 69-70, 80, 86, 94-96, 98-103, 111, 112, 122-124, 129,

Bass Toothbrush 27, 29, 133

Biomimetic 15, 68, 84, 86, 134

Biologic Dentistry . 2-4, 9, 11, 36, 84, 86, 92, 99, 122, 134

Black Beans 55, 56,

Blood Testing 92, 99

Bone Broth 46, 47, 57

Bones 37, 39, 43, 46, 47, 49, 71, 117, 118, 124

Brown Rice 51, 54, 56-57

Brushing Technique 29

Butter 35, 37-40, 48,

Calc Fluor 105, 118

Calc Phos 105, 118

Calcium 17, 28, 35, 37, 39, 42, 43, 45, 46, 49, 51, 59, 96, 103, 104, 117, 118, 124

Cancer 9, 11-13, 27, 37-38, 65, 68, 72, 95, 97, 98, 104, 122, 125, 126

Cavity/Cavitation . 8-10, 15, 19-23, 28-30, 36, 39, 48-49, 51, 60, 62, 68, 70-73, 80, 85, 93, 95, 111-112, 123-124, 127-128

Cementum 16-17, 107

Chocolate Drink 48

Clean 15 . . . . 41-42, 133

Clean and Heal Rinse 32, 33, 105

Cleaning, Mechanical 101

Coconut Sugar 50

Cod Liver Oil 37-38, 48, 133

Cone Beam CT Scan 66

Corn 38, 53, 57-60

Crockpot Chicken 47

Crown 10, 13, 46, 64, 70, 84-86, 91, 107

Dairy 39-40, 42-45, 53

Decay 19-21, 23, 25, 33-35, 37, 39-40, 49, 51, 60, 63, 86, 111-112, 123-124, 129

Deficiency 23, 36, 40, 51, 58, 61, 95, 104, 126

Dental Fluorosis 124-127

Dental Rehabilitation 110

Dental Restorations . . . 15, 77-78, 84-86, 101, 110, 131

Dental Revision 91-92

Dentin 16-17, 19, 22-23, 63, 111

Deprogrammer 109-110

Diabetes 12, 44, 68, 93, 95, 97-98, 126

Diagnostic Testing 99

Diet Theory 20

Digital Xray 14, 66, 68, 70, 111, 119

Dirty Dozen 41-42, 133

Disease 9, 11-12, 19, 23, 26, 33-36, 38, 40, 44, 57-58, 64-68, 72, 79, 93-98, 100-103, 105, 119, 122, 129

Disinfection 63, 69, 72, 102

DNA Testing 99	Infection. 11-13, 18-19, 28, 40, 62-66, 70-71, 91, 93, 95, 98-103, 106, 111, 122
Durathin. 131	
Earthpaste 28, 133	
Enamel 16-17, 19, 21-23, 26, 28, 107, 11-113, 116, 124, 126, 130	Inflammation. . . 50, 62, 94-95, 104, 122, 129
	Jaw Imbalance. 108
Energy Channels. 119-120	Laser 15, 69, 93, 101-102, 111
Environmental Working Group (EWG). . .41, 133	Legumes. 50-55
Fermented Foods. .37, 44-45, 48, 53, 83, 133	Lime Water 58-60
Fillings. 2, 6, 10-11, 13-14, 22, 63-64, 66, 69-71, 73-87, 91, 101, 107, 111, 125, 130	Lipid Panel Test. 99
	Living Granola. 54
	Maple Syrup 50, 115
Fluoride 11, 14, 27, 123-128, 134	Medicine 8, 10-11, 14, 74, 102, 129
Food 3, 5, 10, 20-21, 23, 26, 30-31, 34-61, 80, 83-84, 89-91, 103, 105, 108-109, 112, 115, 118, 120, 125, 128	Mercury 6, 11, 14, 73-86, 101, 130
	Meridian. 90, 119-122
	Metal. 2, 4, 6, 11, 14, 28, 70-71, 74-80, 83, 89-92, 101, 106, 110, 121
Gingivitis 94-96, 100	
Go-Betweens 32, 133	Microbes 18, 41, 44, 61, 70, 72, 93, 99, 102
Grains. 38, 43, 50-54, 91	
Gum Disease. . . 25, 33, 93-94, 101, 103, 105	Minerals 15, 17, 19-21, 28-29, 35-36, 39-40, 43, 49-51, 53, 61, 91, 103, 105, 111-112, 116-118, 123-124, 128, 130
Gum Irrigation. 102	
Gum Tissue 16, 18, 95, 102-103	
Gums, Bleeding. 95-96, 100-104	
HbA1C 99	MouthPaste. 28
Healing 9, 14-15, 32-33, 48, 63, 65, 68-69, 71-72, 84, 92, 102-104, 111	Nutrition 6, 11, 14, 16, 20, 23, 36, 40, 42, 56-57, 60, 68, 91, 93, 95, 99, 103
Heart Disease 9, 12-13, 22, 38-39, 44, 65, 68, 72, 95, 97, 119, 122	Nutritional Counselor, Therapeutic 5-6
	Nuts & Seeds. 38, 45, 51-54
	Oats 53-54, 60
Holistic Dentistry . 1, 3, 6, 8-11, 25, 27, 40, 61, 68, 83-84, 86, 92, 101, 122, 129, 132-133	Oil Pulling. 129-130
	Ozone Cleaning 68-69, 86, 93, 102
Honey. 4-55, 55, 115	Page, Melvin 20, 23,
Hormone Theory 20	Pellegra. 57-58
Horsetail. 117-118	Peridontitis 94-95
IAOMT 74, 78-79, 82, 125-127	Periodontal Disease. 65, 95-98, 100, 102, 122
Imbalance. 23, 101, 108, 122,	
Implant. 2-3, 73, 86-92	Periodontal Ligament 16-17, 71, 94, 96
	Peroxide. 130

Phytates 51, 60,

Phytic Acid. 50-53, 55-56

Plaque. 1-23, 29-31, 42, 90, 94, 96, 100, 102, 117, 122, 129

Price, Westin. 47, 60, 20, 24-36, 40, 49, 51, 64, 66

Pulp. 16-17, 22, 111

Recession, Gum 94, 100, 106-107, 109

Remineralization. . . 15, 28-29, 39, 49, 51, 111-112, 117-118, 124, 128, 130

Research. . . . . 5-8, 11-12, 15, 19-20, 23, 40, 44 ,49, 52, 60, 64-66, 69-72, 77-78, 86, 89, 90, 97, 113, 122-125, 127, 129

Root Canal 3, 9-11, 13, 15, 62-71, 73, 84, 86, 91, 119

Sea Salt. 26, 33, 105, 129

Silica 117-118

Silver. 6, 9, 28, 33

Soaking Grains & Legumes. 52-60

Stevia 28, 50

Stomach 51, 60-61, 68, 117, 122, 128, 130

Sugar. 3, 14, 19-20, 23, 35, 44, 49-50, 55, 60, 91, 95, 99, 103, 112, 114-115, 118

Supplements 5, 36, 39, 41, 46, 61, 83, 103, 105, 117-118, 125, 127-128, 133

Symptoms 4, 10-11, 75, 93, 95, 100-101, 119, 125

Systemic Disease . . .40, 72, 98, 119, 122, 124

Temporo-Mandibular Dysfunction (TMD). . 126,

Temporo-Mandibular Joint (TMJ) 2, 107

Therapeutic IV 92

Titanium Implants. 88-90

Tongue Scraper. 30-31, 105, 133

Tooth Whitening. 129, 130

Toothbrush 10, 23, 27, 29, 105, 107, 129, 133

Toothpaste. 15, 19, 27-29, 116, 123-125, 128, 133

Tortillas. 59

Toxic-Toxin 2, 6, 9, 11, 15, 18, 20, 26-28, 58, 63, 65, 71-72, 74-75, 77, 83, 90-92, 94, 96, 122, 124-126

Treatment. 11, 13, 27-28, 62, 64, 66, 68-69,75, 81, 83, 91-93, 97, 99, 101-103, 105, 109-110, 119

Umbrella Effect. 21

Veneers 131

Vitamin D3 Test 92

Vitamins 35-36, 38-40, 42-43, 47-51, 57-58, 61, 91-92, 95, 99, 101, 103-105, 117-118, 130

Voll, Reinhold 11-12, 120

Water Irrigation 32, 102-103

Waterpik 32

Western Medicine 10

Whole-Body 9, 11, 12, 15, 84, 135, 137

Zirconium Implants 88-89

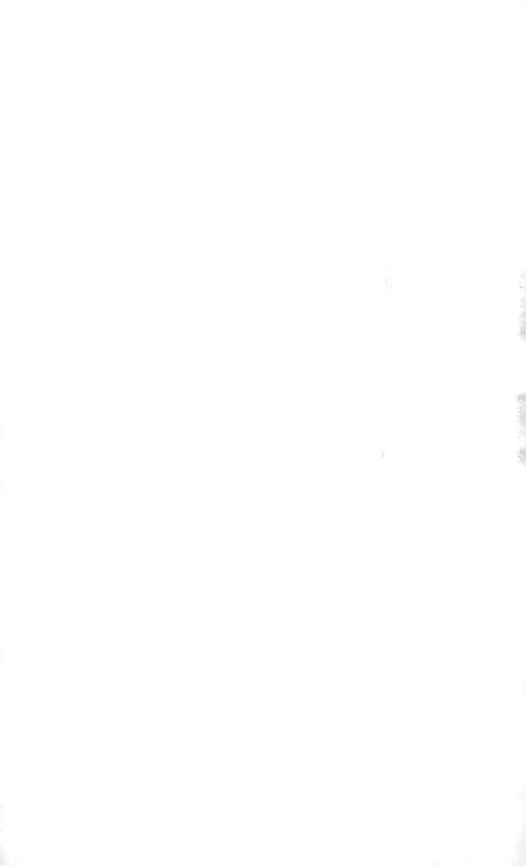

Made in the USA
Middletown, DE
15 July 2019